MEDICAL ROBOTS
Are Accepting New Patients

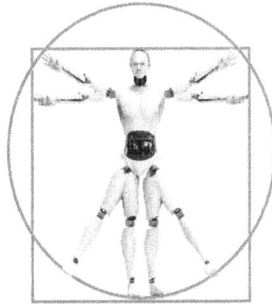

James W. Forsythe, M.D., H.M.D.

Contents

Dedication

This book is dedicated to my grandchildren and future great-grandchildren, the pivotal generations that represent humanity's future survival amid a world filled with medical robots.

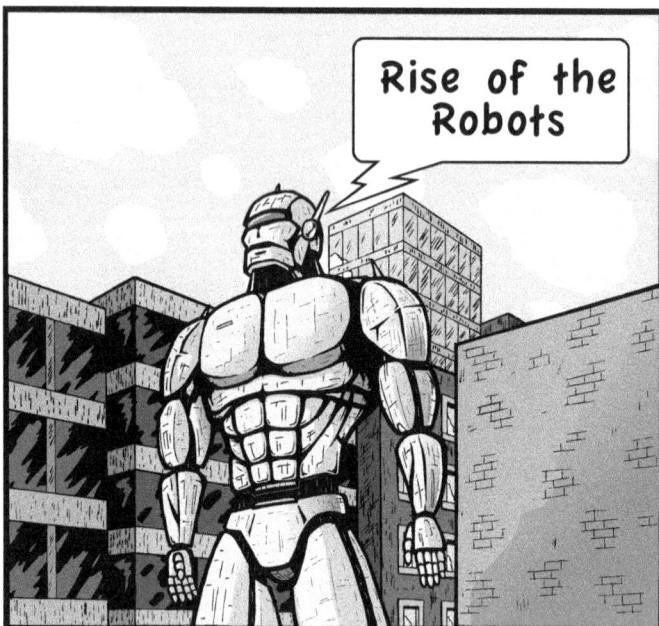

Chapter 1
Introducing Medical Robots

Machines will rule your body.

Yes, mechanical devices determine whether you live or die.

And, no, this is far from a make-believe world.

Virtually all of mankind will change as a result.

Like this or not, from the moment new babies are born until the day they die, hopefully in old age, virtually all of them will have their bodies monitored by machines.

Disturbing Transition Sweeps the World

This highly disturbing transition is well underway.

Virtually unnoticed by the vast majority of us, the medical robotics industry is on the verge of changing how everyone lives and dies.

Some people might call this the "Rise of the Robots" or the "Rise of Machines."

Whatever words are used to label this rapidly accelerating trend, the international transition has become unstoppable.

Just as disturbing, this overall change is "real" rather than mere science fiction.

A Nightmare Has Become Reality

Until this point, the mainstream news media has ignored this issue.

That is why you very likely have heard little--if anything--about this universal transition until now.

Right off the bat, there are two critical underlying factors that you need to learn.

First, this transition is all about you, focused primarily on your overall health for as long as you're alive.

Then, there's a second urgent factor, namely the relationship between you and your real, live human physician. Yet will that doctor-patient relationship gradually deteriorate, as robots steadily replace people who have medical expertise?

This Transition Boggles the Mind

A fast-moving and unstoppable transition within the entire healthcare industry looms above us all in this regard. The average person likely becomes mentally numb upon first learning these details, which dive deep into the core of "what it means to be human."

To help put the transition into clear perspective, think of the situation this way: Right now medical robotics are at a developmental stage, the technological equivalent of the early 1990s amid the Rise of the Internet.

As almost everyone knows today, by early in this century the online world had begun to virtually rule, regulate and control the successes, failures and advances in human relationships and in business.

The Web's dominance in our personal lives and industry has evolved into an "accepted fact," a stunning transition when considering that just a few decades ago most people lacked any knowledge about the online world. In the early 1990s, the development and initial building of the Web's infrastructure was well underway, although only a relatively small percentage of the public knew.

Everything changed considerably by the last few years of that decade, when huge percentages of the population had finally gravitated online.

Seemingly within the blink of an eye, the basic building blocks of the Internet began to assist, regulate and control seemingly every aspect of business, communication, and social interaction.

Face This Disturbing Reality Head-On

At this pivotal juncture, humanity finds itself ensconced in the equivalent of the early 1990s as far as any comparison between the birth of the Internet and today's advancements in medical robotics.

With this clearly understood, the situation becomes somewhat disturbing when considering the fact that most doctors today fail to realize what is about to occur.

These medical professionals need to know as soon as possible that in all likelihood, the entire medical industry will change at a rapid-fire pace. Doctors, nurses and hospital personnel will finally discover that robots are being created to take their jobs.

With equal intensity, today's medical professionals become emotionally stunned upon discovering these inescapable facts; major corporations are steadily pushing this transition into overdrive on an international scale.

Shockingly, unless decisive action reverses this trend soon, the decision-making process regarding health care could be ripped away from humans--as medical robotic-devices begin making "life-and-death choices for patients."

Calm Down and Accept the Cold-Hard Facts

This might sound bizarre to read or to say in any regard. But the following is undeniable.

Before long, a robot--a mere machine--likely will have the ability and the authorization to determine whether you live or you die.

Of course, to almost any sound, sane and reasonably intelligent person today, such a revelation might seem bizarre and downright "other-worldly."

Without question, the mere mention of this inescapable transition triggers proverbial alarm bells within the minds of rational-thinking people.

Yet as you will soon learn in full unabridged detail, scientists, electrical engineers and major corporations worldwide are well along in the process of making this occur.

You Are Their Target

As if these revelations were not already enough to cause earthquakes within the human psyche, you, your family and virtually everyone that you know are their proverbial "targets."

The so-called "humanity factor" is about to get ripped out of the entire medical industry as this wide-scale change clicks into full gear.

In a sense, you are directly within the "cross-hairs" of major corporations worldwide that plan to to use robots to regulate, control and administer health care.

You see, these robots, mechanical devices and automated digital systems are already in the mid- and even-late development phases.

The rollout of these machines into every aspect of the medical industry is planned on a step-by-step scheduled, set to rapidly accelerate during the next decade and beyond.

A "Disturbing Future" Looms

Like this or not, these disturbing transitions have already begun.

In fact, if this trend holds as steady as some medical industry analysts predict, by the mid-2020s medical robots will be considered necessary and vital to medical care.

Then, by the end of that decade into the mid-2030s, robots and automated machinery will gradually control and operate almost every aspect of the healthcare industry.

Powerful enough to rattle the "proverbial soul" of humanity, this new infrastructure will monitor, control and even regulate the health of each human being.

"That is ludicrous!" many people might understandably exclaim when first learning this. "How could such a thing possibly happen! This is all pure fantasy."

Chapter 2
The Inescapable Reality

You must accept these grim facts.

You need to do so because there is no way to escape.

First and foremost, envision the end-phase of your life, hopefully in old age.

Up to now, the vast majority of us who think at least briefly about the end-phase of our lives envision being surrounded by relatives when the end comes.

With any luck, leading up to your hoped-for peaceful demise, in those final days a caring human doctor and perhaps nurses would handle all of your basic needs.

To the contrary, though, when your "time comes," in all likelihood, if you pass away from slowly progressing natural causes sometime after 2030, you in all likelihood will be surrounded by robots and machines rather than human doctors and nurses.

Human Doctors Become Rare

Perhaps most disturbing, at least from the perspective of most people, by some point within that transitional period *you will be lucky if you ever get to see a real-live human doctor*.

Such a maddening situation becomes exacerbated when taking into account the inescapable fact that the U.S. government wants you to die at home surrounded by robotic health-monitoring devices--rather than perish in a hospital or hospice.

Under the Affordable Health Care Act, the travesty commonly known as "Obamacare," the vast majority of people older than 80 will be confined to their homes during their final years--rather than in overcrowded senior care facilities.

A primary reason for this mandate required by the ill-conceived and inefficient regulations stems from the fact that the older senior population is "literally busting at the seams" as Baby

Boomers reach retirement and advanced age.

As if to poke a proverbial dagger into the heart of this issue, our politicians and the bureaucrats who kowtow to them have devilishly devised a system mandating the use of robotic or automatic health-monitoring systems within home environments.

Human Doctors Become an "Endangered Species"

This is not intended as any kind of crude joke or exaggeration whatsoever. The inescapable truth remains that real-live human doctors may soon become the equivalent of the spotted owl--an endangered species on the verge of extinction.

To make such a proclamation understandably might seem outlandish or even foolish. After all, how in heaven's name could such a situation occur?

Well, to tell you the truth, scientists actually are well along in the process of conceiving, designing, developing and "rolling out" machines that serve as physicians.

From the perspective of most of us "mere humans," that concept is "way out there," far from the realm possibility. The mere notion of replacing doctors with machines strikes people as develish, inhuman and "literally unthinkable."

Even the futuristic science fiction "Star Trek" TV and film series that began in the 1960s featured a human physician nicknamed "Bones" rather than a robotic doctor. Many of that series' once-futuristic gadgets have subsequently become "reality," particularly wireless phones that enable humans to communicate "through the sky."

The rapidly approaching advancement of medical robotics has emerged as perhaps the one thing that "Star Trek" creator Gene Roddenberry failed to predict.

Understand My Unique Perspective

Now in my fifth decade as a practicing physician, I have earned a positive international reputation as a practitioner of standard and alternative natural medicine.

These are among key factors giving me a unique perspective into primary issues involving health care and urgent medical industry trends.

Determined to meet strong public demand for my knowledge, I have written dozens of books, read daily by consumers and doctors worldwide.

Largely as a result, people view me as an international leader in giving them vital medical industry updates, in many cases urgent details that are otherwise difficult to find.

This book is the result of bursting consumer demand, perhaps the first publication of its kind designed to give common people everywhere the truth about medical robotics.

Discover This Inescapable Truth

The vast majority of my books until now have been the result of patients and consumers urging me to reveal the truth about medical issues. My previous topics have covered a vast array of challenges, ranging from anti-cancer diets to medical marijuana.

This publication marks an all-new pathway in my burgeoning array of books, now numbering more than 20.

You see, I pride myself in keeping up with all the latest technologies designed to improve health.

Along the way, thanks partly to my research assistants, I discovered what until now has been the little-known but vital issue of medical robotics.

Once I found out a handful of these startling details, I launched an intense research project into this essential topic, which until the publication of this book has largely been ignored by the mainstream media.

People Look to Me for Leadership

At this point, you might wonder, "What makes Doctor Forsythe such an expert on this issue? Why should I pay any attention to him?"

Well, one factor setting me apart from all "the rest of the pack" is that I'm an "integrative medical oncologist," among just a handful of such medical professionals in the USA.

Thanks to this unique and powerful designation, I have the rare ability to practice medicine as a standard allopathic or "mainstream" oncologist, while also integrating natural medicines into treatment.

In the process, I have developed an advanced Stage IV cancer treatment protocol that generates nearly 33 times better results than the national average.

Understandably as a result, every week patients from around the world stream to my Century Wellness Clinic in Reno, Nevada, in the western United States.

Patients Express Dismay

During the final few months before this book's initial release, I occasionally chatted with a handful of my friends about the coming massive change engulfing the healthcare industry due to robotics.

"What in the world!" one person exclaimed. "This sounds preposterous! You mean to tell me that robots are going to help run or manage the medical industry?"

When I respond by giving in-depth detail, these people invariably confess to their personal dismay, anger and frustration with this destructive situation. At a rapidly accelerating pace, these technological developments in medical robotics leave many consumers feeling perplexed and somewhat hopeless.

Motivated at least in part on this unscientific personal survey, I intensified my research into this vital and inescapable issue.

In the pages that follow, I suspect that you likely will become equally frustrated and concerned, particularly upon learning more about this increasingly critical situation.

Most Doctors Lack Information

Every step of the way in this learning process, keep in mind that as previously stated, upon this book's initial publication most doctors lacked any inkling of the coming massive international change impacting the entire healthcare industry.

Like clockwork for many decades I have attended numerous annual medical industry seminars, where physicians and scientists share urgent information on big medical discoveries.

In all that time, never once have I seen presentations or read reports at such gatherings on the fast-approaching industry-wide change generated by robotics.

This brings up numerous questions that deserve answers, namely why and how the vast majority of doctors and medical professionals have been "kept in the dark."

As you'll soon discover, the overall situation is far from a mere conspiracy theory, but rather the result of rapid technological advancements.

Stand Up for Your Rights

After much intense research, I have concluded that at the heart of this issue rests the critical relationship between doctors and their patients.

People can and should become understandably angry when discovering these details, which for the most part--like I say--have been kept from the public until now.

Why in the world would any person ever want or agree to put his or her life "in the hands of a mere machine, with no human doctor present?"

Perhaps just as critical comes the question: "Why would physicians, medical facilities and electrical engineers ever agree to such a massive transition?"

With equal intensity, how or why should consumers allow these changes to click into full gear, to a point where the trend becomes unstoppable?

Get Critical Details

The answers to these questions disturb me, just as I suspect they will leave you perplexed as well.

For these reasons, I'm about to "map out" all these various factors in full detail, giving much of the information in a matter-of-fact way for your careful consideration.

Along the way, you will discover precisely how, when and where these changes in robotics will change the patient experience in most aspects of the medical industry.

As a result, you will learn how this new technology will impact patients, from the moment they check in to hospitals or medical facilities, until check-out time.

In the process, you'll also discover how patients will be expected to behave in order to regain optimal health.

Consider Patient Outcomes

With equal intensity, you need my personal analysis on whether these machines will eventually have an ability to generate short- and long-term diagnosis for patients.

Adding another critical aspect, you also will get my unique perspective on how the addition of robotics will impact patient costs.

In addition, taking this a logical step further, you can look forward to my perspective on how all this will change the entire medical industry.

You also need to know why researchers and electrical engineers likely will want to block any efforts that you might make to stop this disturbing transition.

Needless to say, I feel a burning need to give you these critical details that some officials might want to censor or withhold from the public. Yes, while some politicians and government bureaucrats might argue otherwise, consumers can and should have a right to know the truth--cognizant that widespread publicity on the medical robotics issue has been relatively scant until now.

Similar attention needs to go to existing doctors,

prospective physicians and all other medical industry professionals.

Just as much as the patients, such individuals have a right to know at this early juncture what will be expected of them amid the "Rise of the Robots" into the healthcare industry and elsewhere throughout society.

Putting even more angst into the potential brew, "human doctors," nurses, and even hospital cleaning crews need to know robotics will endanger their jobs.

As if all this were not already enough to cause intense concern, you'll also discover the likely impact of healthcare robots on medical schools and scientific research.

Ultimately, these converging factors likely will bring about an intense quest by the general public to "keep humanity--to keep people--in the equation at all times."

Understand My Unique Perspective

From this point forward, you will receive my no-holds-barred perspective on these essential and interlinking issues--which likely will change humanity forevermore.

Think of this as a "for the better or for the worse" situation, somewhat similar to traditional wedding vows.

While the overall transition signals that "there can be no turning back," you'll also get my viewpoint on how to prevent the process from damaging humanity.

By using the term "humanity" in this regard, I mean the heart, soul and God-given personality of every person on earth.

Yes, people have a right and even a responsibility to live apart from machines, without having to rely on robots to remain alive.

Public Reports Prove Vital

Once again, and this is well-worth stating, I cannot possibly begin to emphasize enough that my analysis and all the cutting-edge details you will find in the pages that follow are based on news reports, corporate press releases and scientific research.

The vast majority of these news stories get relatively little publicity, probably viewed by most average people as a "mere curiosity, mostly forgettable."

As of the time of this book's initial publication, a smattering of sporadic news stories had chronicled everything from remote surgeries performed via robots to new machines used to clean and sanitize hospital rooms.

For the most part, these various advancements were touted as mere curiosities. Yet if the truth be told, the devices marked the beginning of a massive transition into fully digitalized, robotic, and hospital-based drug delviery systems worldwide.

Rather than reveal how hospitals will drastically change, for the most part the news media has chosen to portray the overall situation as if a "far-out scientific fantasy."

Chapter 3
Medical Transformations Engulf the Earth

The medical industry transition will rapidly change the experiences of everyone needing urgent medical attention, at least based on published news reports and robotics advancements announced by corporations and university research programs.

With these reports as a model, here are typical medical response, treatment and rehabilitation scenarios. The following hypothetical examples are listed separately for the years 2025 and 2035, each listed differently due to expected advancements in robotics.

Under the following hypothetical scenario, you have been seriously injured in the crash of a helicopter that smashed into a vacant parking lot near a busy freeway--about 10 miles from the nearest major city. The accident happened at 5:24 in the late afternoon, amid rush-hour on a Wednesday.

You are the only survivor from among four people who were riding in the helicopter. The three other people died instantly upon impact.

You lost consciousness due to massive head trauma. Your only other serious injury is a severe gouging wound on your upper leg above the left knee. This results in severe bleeding that, if left untreated, will result in your death.

Initial Response Action

An automated signaling device within the aircraft, a so-called updated "black box system," immediately notifies authorities that the crash has occurred.

The instant data communication system gives authorities the location, time and severity of the mishap. The initial response by police, firefighters and the medical team begins full-force within 10 seconds after the accident.

2025: All the current modern emergency vehicles are self-driving machines, and by this point at least 85 percent to 95 percent of all cars on U.S. highways have these systems. Even so, the average emergency response time during 2025 is still several minutes, largely because the roads remain clogged with vehicles that require humans to take over steering chores in order to pull over to the side of the highway. While en route, emergency personnel lack any information on the number and severity of injuries, if any.

2035: The emergency response team takes less than two or three minutes. Thanks to updated technology, all civilian vehicles instantly pull to the side of effected roads and highways, clearing the way for emergency vehicles. This improved system enables police, fire and medical units to zip at more than 90 miles per hour to the accident scene. For you, this is a crucial benefit, since super-fast medical response times sharply increase the probability that officials will be able to save you.

Accident Scene Assessment

Adhering to standard "emergency services protocol" that has been universally used since at least the 1950s, authorities strive to quickly assess damage, any danger to property and the severity of injuries to each victim.

2025: Upon arriving on scene, human firefighters risk their lives if necessary to suppress any fire or to neutralize any fuel spillage that might otherwise lead to a possible explosion. Meantime, human police officers secure the area to prevent unauthorized people from entering the danger zone. Even so, although at this point all vehicles have self-driving systems, curious humans are able to take over steering or to slow down their vehicles--in a somewhat voyeuristic desire to "rubber-neck" and gaze at the wreckage. This jams traffic as curious people slow down on nearby freeways or roads; some onlookers attempt to drive to the scene to get a closer look. Most important for you, human paramedics use the latest machines to assess your overall physical condition and bodily vital signs. This essential information is automatically sent to human doctors and various highly trained medical professionals, all gathered in the Emergency Room of the licensed hospital located in the city. Based on the data, these doctors give the human paramedics specific orders on how to administer your initial treatment on scene and--if necessary--to try to stabilize your vital signs.

2035: As required by law, indestructible robots already were on board with the people before the helicopter crashed. Within 30 to 45 seconds after the mishap, these undamaged robots have fully assessed the severity of injuries to all people on board. Amazingly, just one minute after the accident, thanks to the robots and instant communications, the "doctors" at the city hospital already know every basic detail of your physical condition. The vast majority of physicians at the hospital are not people, but rather robots--sometimes called "RoboDocs." Also, by this point, the world's self-driving vehicles and the overall transportation system has been significantly improved. Because your personal information and health history have been input into a national database, the machines at the emergency room already know your entire medical history. About 90 seconds after the crash, automated communication systems have begun to notify your relatives; they receive details of the crash and your condition. In all likelihood, most or all of the arriving paramedics are robots, although some humans might be involved as well. With luck, by the time firefighters arrive on scene, any fire or fuel spillage has already been suppressed or at least somewhat contained by the robots that were on the helicopter.

Medical Transport

As indicated earlier, super-fast medical response and patient-transportation times sharply increase an accident victim's probability of survival.

2025: On average nationwide, thanks partly to advances in robotics, average ambulance response times are significantly better than just one decade earlier in 2015. However, while authorities attempt to rush you to the hospital, the operators of most self-driving cars must personally take over operation of their vehicles in order to steer to the side of roadways. Just as is the case today, upon hearing sirens drivers will be required to move their vehicles to the right in order to clear a pathway for emergency vehicles approaching from behind. This will slow your arrival at the hospital somewhat, because most of the time while traveling in their "self-driving cars" on freeways and surface streets, people "behind the wheel" pay little or no attention to the operation of their vehicles. The sound of sirens will interrupt the human motorists from reading, watching TV or even sleeping in their moving cars, in order for these people to slow down and steer their vehicles to the side. Meantime, while en route to the hospital, the human paramedics use machines to improve or stabilize your vital signs while en route to the hospital. Also, just as is the case today for the most part, in keeping with established medical industry protocol, these paramedics strive to refrain from performing any physically intrusive procedures while still in the ambulance. If necessary, however, they occasionally use essential emergency medical techniques, such as applying a tourniquet to cut off or suppress blood flow from your leg wound; this is done to prevent excessive bleeding and possible death.

2035: The time needed to transport you to the hospital is seemingly "lightning-fast" from the human perspective, thanks to the updated technology that forces all self-driving cars to the side of roadways to clear the way for emergency vehicles. These movements will happen automatically, without the guidance of human drivers in each vehicle. Remember that most or all of the "paramedics" at this point are actually robots; these machines either look, behave and move precisely like humans. This is done by design in order to prevent people from becoming confused or overly afraid. While en route to the hospital you still remain unconscious due to severe head trauma. Although transportation time lasts just several minutes at most, there is a possibility that the on-board paramedic machines might "choose" to perform a surgical procedure on you while still on board. Even before leaving the accident scene, the paramedics have sent a Cat-Scan image of your head via the Internet; the images would be received by human doctors or RoboDocs in the Emergency Room as they await your arrival. Any decision on whether to operate while still in the ambulance would be almost instant. If deemed necessary, while still in the ambulance the paramedic-robots could attempt to remove a portion of your skull. Even today, such procedures are sometimes done, but only in hospitals many hours after accidents. The skull-removal procedures are done in order to prevent swelling of the brain from causing a potentially fatal build-up of pressure within the head. Also, during transport in 2035, if your leg wound continues to bleed, rather than use an "old-fashioned tourniquet," robotic paramedics at the accident scene or inside the ambulance would have the ability to use lasers to cauterize the wound. This would be an attempt to instantly stop bleeding, decreasing chances of shock.

In-Hospital Preparations

Just as is the case today, under these near-future scenarios, while the ambulance is en route, hospital personnel will make all necessary preparations to receive you as a patient. This will happen whether the medical facility "workers" are robots or people.

2025: During the final few minutes before your arrival, human doctors and nurses use antiseptic soap and hot water to clean their hands and arms. Also, following standard procedures that have been employed for many decades, the operating room setting has been hand-scrubbed in advance of your arrival at the operating room. At this point in rare instances, devices using infrared lights disinfect these medical professionals, the entire room and all surgical devices. Meantime, a highly skilled human surgeon is already on standby if necessary to operate on you--but in most instances there is a significant variation from procedures conducted as little as 10 years earlier in 2015. Back then, some human doctors still performed such surgeries in person. However, by this juncture in 2025, most surgeries of this nature are handled remotely by human physicians who are physically at a facility other than hospital where you are located. To perform "telesurgery," the human surgeon puts his or her hands inside a mechanical device. In this example, the human surgeon is in Chicago, while you are in Atlanta. While this is happening, the surgeon looks into a computer screen to see TV-style images of your body--specifically the area of your wound. Simultaneously, a mechanical device is inside the operating room beside you. Thanks to this instantaneous Internet communication, by moving his hands the surgeon is able to control and to manipulate the surgical machines that are beside your body in the operating room. While controlled by the surgeon, the device cuts into your body. Under this scenario, the initial operation is done on your head because physicians have deemed this wound is by far the most severe, life-threatening of your two injuries.

    2035: In many scenarios, chances are extremely high that the "physician" operating on you is actually a robot. This is the case, whether the surgery is done "in-person" or remotely as described in the 2025 example. One of the spookiest and most surreal aspects of these 2035 surgeries is the fact that robots performing the operations are "autonomous;" robots with these duties are programmed to make their own spontaneous decisions. These life-or-death choices will be made on what people call "the spur-of-the moment," fluid situations where conditions typically change often. So, like people do, the surgical RoboDoc continually analyzes your physical condition amid the surgery. All along, the robots are programmed to do everything reasonably possible to save you, striving to maintain or enhance your overall quality of your life.

    At this early juncture, now in the 2010s, it's too early to predict whether the surgical robots will be programmed to experience or display "emotion"--or whether electrical engineers will design the machines to behave as if "emotionally cold and heartless."

Hospital Admission Process

Somewhat similar to today's hospital systems, most or all major medical facilities amid the 2020s and 2030s will have strict protocol for admitting patients. In steadily progressing phases by that point, the facilities will have drastically different procedures than those commonplace today.

2025: Immediately prior to your arrival by ambulance at the hospital, your admission forms will already be ready. Assuming that you remain unconscious, doctors assisted by robotic or automated systems will already have an initial treatment protocol for your short- and long-term treatment. If necessary in the event that you remain too ill to sign any forms, your relatives might be requested to authorize that physicians commence with necessary treatments.

2035: Before your arrival at the hospitals, based on the latest technology of that time--coupled with the medical industry's experiences treating previous patients with similar injuries--your "physicians" will have listed your chances for survival on a percentage basis. Just as essential, authorities will estimate your projected treatment time in the facility, plus specific tasks needed to help ensure your survival and rehabilitation.

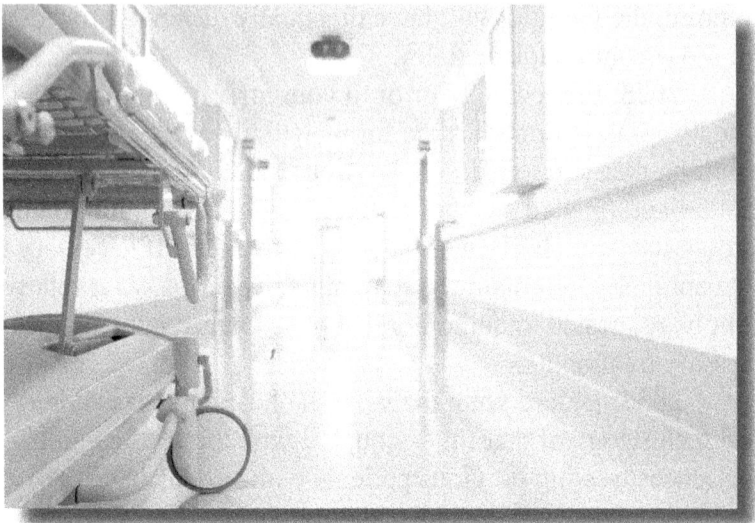

Chapter 4
The Hospital Experience Evolves

Especially from the perspective of anyone born before 1990, the overall experience of being a patient or a visitor at a hospital will seem "other-worldly."

People aged 35 or older likely will feel as if they have entered a science fiction movie, perhaps commenting to each other, "Boy, things have changed."

To humans who have been healthcare professionals for many years by the mid-2020s, these transformations will seem to have been relatively methodical.

Most of these industry-wide changes will not occur "all at once," but rather in a step-by-step process, done in well-planned phases.

Because they will have no other choice, the vast majority of healthcare industry employees will accept and embrace these transitions into their work processes.

Job Losses Anticipated

Although the employees will initially embrace these administrative and procedural changes, gradually most humans working in the hospital industry will lose their jobs. Tasks that the humans once performed will be taken over by robots.

These job losses will mirror a trend first predicted in 2015 by the prestigious "Business Insider" magazine. The publication quoting robotics experts and business analysts who predicted that 47 percent of all workers nationwide would lose their jobs to robots by the early 2030s.

From the perspective of human employees in every industry, the long-term outlook is even gloomier; these disturbing employment forecasts are largely based on an urgent warning issued jointly in 2015 by several of the world's most respected business leaders and scientists.

Those who courageously predicted that virtually all human

jobs will eventually be taken by robots included: billionaire Bill Gates, the founder of Microsoft; Stephen Hawking, an internationally acclaimed physicist; Elon Musk, a world-famous entrepreneur; and Stephen "Steve" Wozniak, a legendary initial developer of Apple Computers.

These luminaries were among a steadily growing list of technology experts who individually and collectively predicted that robots would eventually dominate or even control every profession.

Society Remained Oblivious

Despite such forecasts, as of 2016, the vast majority of people throughout society either remained oblivious to the coming change in hospitals--or in denial.

As previously mentioned, most doctors at that point remained unaware that these changes were about to engulf their industry.

Perhaps such ignorance is to be expected. After all, most people seem to balk at the concept of such wide-scale change.

By early 2016 the overall transition was well underway although a huge percentage of society remained oblivious to the ongoing robotics research and development.

Yet, as previously mentioned, anyone who paid attention to sporadic news stories, corporate press releases and research reports would have known otherwise.

Notice These Changes

The entire hospital experience of the near future will seem foreign or at least vastly different from today, at least judging by forecasts made by robotics professionals from the 2010s.

Assuming that those predictions hold true, here is a general timeline and description of the process--using the same years as in the previous chapter.

2025: Robots and mechanical devices play a key role in the operation and maintenance of almost every hospital.

2035: In a major leap from just a decade earlier, robots and robotic machines play a dominant role in caring for patients and also controlling medical facility operations.

As a result of these transitions, a vast majority or--shockingly--even almost all human employees of the facilities will have their jobs eliminated. Among those losing their positions, usually in phases as robots enter the workplace, will be:

Nurses: These healthcare professionals will not be replaced immediately, but rather in phases over a lengthy period of time. Rather than relying on humans, hospitals will use machines to administer drugs to patients and to monitor their vital signs.

Staffers: Admission clerks, secretaries and phone answering personnel will find their jobs filled by robots at a much faster pace than nurses.

Cleaning crews: Robots will handle all facility maintenance duties, from cleaning patient rooms and scrubbing hallways, to collecting and disposing of trash.

Administration: With steadily increased emphasis, robotic or computer-based systems will help the hospitals' human executives make administrative decisions.

Timeline for Hospitals

Using the examples already listed , the following are examples of what patients and their families should expect at most hospitals.

2025: Patients and visitors benefit from interaction with human employees of the hospital, particularly nurses, admissions personnel and doctors. By this point machines or software programs have eliminated some jobs, while assisting almost all human personnel who remain.

2035: Increasingly frustrated human patients and their families understandably become somewhat disturbed because most or all hospital "personnel" are robots.

In an effort to rectify or "cover-up" this problem, the need for real-life human interaction, some or all hospitals will use use humanoids. Remember, these are machines that look and behave as if "real humans." By 2016 scientists had already made significant advancements in creating new technology necessary for developing machines idential to people.

Hospital Rounds

As far back as 2014, a limited number of hospitals worldwide were already using rather crude robotic devices to help "make the rounds" in visiting patient rooms.

Human doctors have been making the rounds in hospitals for centuries, visiting patients in order to monitor their conditions, make diagnosis and manage treatments.

The initial foray of robotics into this realm began by using crude machines that traveled on rollers somewhat similar to tank tracks. Used in hundreds of hospitals worldwide by 2016, these devices are called "telepresence robots."

These machines are controlled by actual physicians. For instance, a doctor sitting in Barcelona, Spain, might "do the rounds" at a hospital in London, England.

The doctor controls a hand-held device that regulates movements of the machine. In addition, the physician has a chart or computer-generated printout of the patient's physical condition and vital signs.

From the patient's perspective, if the person remains awake and fully cognizant of the surrounding environment, the telepresence robot can be seen entering the Emergency Room or patient room. On the machine is a small TV screen, upon which the patient sees a live image of the human doctor's face.

And from the human doctor's viewpoint, a remote video-cam image of the patient can be seen in the room; the "real-live human" doctor in this example is in Spain.

While viewing remote images of each other, the patient and the doctor chat about the patient's condition, progress and expected treatment. Also, if the patient's relatives are in the room they can join in the discussion.

Patient Interaction Evolves Drastically

In the rounds process, the interaction between patient and doctor is likely to change dramatically in the years used in our examples:

2025: Almost every hospital uses robotic devices with video screens to complete patient rounds, unlike just ten years ago when only a small percentage of such facilities used or allowed the devices. Yet by this point, the communication systems and video images have been dramatically improved. At least one significant change involves the human doctor's ability to touch the patient's body using a robotic arm. This is done when the human physician manipulates a device that regulates the robot's movement. From hundreds or even thousands of miles away, the doctor can "feel" or at least sense the actual reaction or condition of the patient's body.

2035: In all likelihood by this point, or around 2040 at the latest, some or all of the doctors "who do the rounds" are humanoids. One of the scariest aspects of this transition is the inescapable fact that many or all of the robots will be "fully autonomous." This means that the robots operate independent and separate from humans. Gone are the days from just a decade or so earlier when human doctors--working in conjunction with robots--played a critical, essential and necessary role in each interaction with a patient.

The Elimination of Human Doctors

For obvious reasons, this potential elimination of human doctors will emerge as the "hot-button issue." Angry, frustrated and afraid for a good reason, people are likely to balk or even to protest that the prospect of whether they live or die would be "put into the artificial hands of mere machines."

When and if this unfathomable transition occurs, for the most part most consumers will find themselves left with no option other than to "follow these orders."

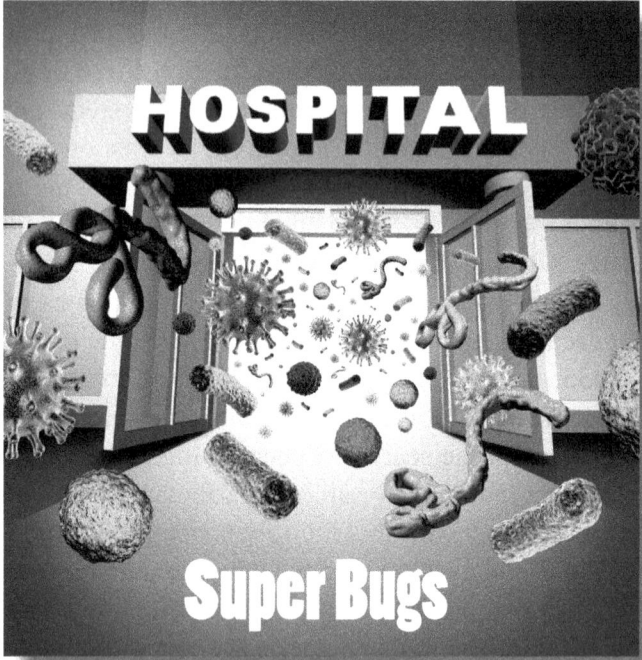

Chapter 5
Medical Environments Change

If the overall transitions occur in the form and timeline that many analysts predict, the environment and culture of virtually every hospital will drastically change.

On an overall basis, these transitions supposedly will improve the care and long-term outcome of most average patients.

While such a system obviously has yet to prove itself as effective, electrical engineers and scientists remain busy planning these transitions.

"This is a landmark evolution in medical technology that will improve the quality and efficiency of health care for as long as humans exist," some observers might say. "Before long, the standard hospital environments typical today will seem antiquated."

Even so, there remain those of us who are highly skeptical at the mere thought of such a transformation. We warn, "Be careful what you ask for, largely because a hellish situation could very well erupt--primarily the potential loss of human hospital employees from the equation."

Cleanliness and Godliness

For many generations, doctors and medical professionals have realized the extreme importance of a critial, essential and non-stop need to maintain and clean medical environments-- hopefully making those areas germ-free .

Yet in recent years well into the 2010s, news stories have regularly chronicled "superbugs" that enter hospital and sicken many people.

Until now, the failure of hospitals to implement efficient antiseptic environments has been the key instigator of such critical problems.

However, the potential danger to patients has worsened

significantly due to the advent of viruses that have become immune to powerful antibiotics.

From the viewpoint of scientists and medical professionals, superbugs pose extreme danger, even within the so-called everyday environment outside of hospitals and medical clinics.

Robotics Come to the Rescue?

If all goes as planned, robotics will come to the rescue. Working non-stop, the machines will be designed to continually eradicate hospitals of all germs.

This transition is supposed to click into gear in stepped phases, steadily improving as healthcare facilities adopt and integrate robotic technology. With persistence, these devices should become fully operational by the early to mid-2020s. In fact, many of these changes already are underway in several U.S. hospitals.

As previously mentioned, an ultimate goal is to eliminate human cleaning crews, largely because people are deemed unreliable, while lacking machine-like efficiency. Among the changes or benefits envisioned by the robotics industry:

Patient rooms: Several times daily, robots using ultraviolet lights and scrubbers fully clean each patient room in the entire hospital. The devices travel automatically from room to room, completing tasks even while patients, visitors or medical professionals are present. Barely noticed by humans due to their quiet and efficient operations, the machines fully clean and disinfect every square centimeter of the entire room. The efficient disinfection occurs on the floors, walls and ceilings, plus any adjoining restroom. Assuming that the technology progresses as planned, the average cleaning time for an individual patient room will be about three minutes. Several of these "cleaning robots" on each patient floor will perform their tasks on a 24-hour basis.

Public areas: Robots that continually clean all public areas of the hospital including hallways, doors and elevators will have the same function as the machines that clean patient rooms. Yet public-area machines have a significantly different design. Somewhat larger than patient-room robots, these devices also use ultraviolet light.

Air scrubbers: Machines that continually clean the air also become necessary, because germs and particularly superbugs become airborne--rather than merely landing on surfaces. Like the patient-room and public-area cleaning machines, the air scrubbers will continually patrol and disinfect the entire hospital. Before the self-moving air scrubbers get developed and implemented, many healthcare facilities are likely to use non-movable or stationary air filtering devices.

Refuse disposal: As previously mentioned, automated or robotic devices will continually dispose of trash from the entire facility. This is an especially critical chore because some garbage generated at hospitals contains papers or devices that are contaminated with extremely dangerous viruses. In all likelihood, the trash-collecting robots also will use ultraviolet lights to disinfect the garbage beginning at the moment the machine collects the materials. Then the machines will zip to a garbage-disposal room inside the facility, or to a a pre-designated area outside the structure. At these zones where humans are prohibited for safety reasons, machines efficiently compress or squeeze the unwanted substances. This new garbage-removal process eliminates potential danger to humans inside the entire hospital. Another long-term goal will involve recycling; this entails what the term implies, gathering temporarily discarded materials that can be re-used or recycled. At least by some accounts, recycling will become increasingly critical on an international scale, as humans everywhere strive to use robots to enhance the environment; this is done to minimize or eliminate any degradation to the ecosystem.

Pharmaceutical Distribution
By most accounts, the future prescribing, distribution and

administration of drugs in hospitals will seem "far out," a pure fantasy or a goofy science fiction plot.

Yet these changes in hospital pharmacology will occur on a widespread scale if scientists and electrical engineers become successful with their current research and development efforts.

In almost every instance today, highly trained and educated people operate pharmacies within hospitals. As of the time of this book's publication, only a handful of those operations were fully automated. The current transition involves prescriptions issued by human physicians that serve patients in healthcare facilities.

In the vast majority of instances, right now the drugs are distributed in two primary ways, with a limited number of exceptions. First, some hospital pharmacies fulfill prescription orders to patients who have just been checked out of the facility.

The second and most common modern in-hospital pharmacy distribution involves hospital employees who deliver the prescribed pharmaceuticals to patient rooms, general care areas such as Intensive Care Units (ICUs), and operating rooms.

Today's human-based hospital pharmacies require efficiency on a broad scale, largely because of these wide-ranging duties and responsibilities. Yet "human error" sometimes occurs, due the huge volume of orders for drugs.

By contrast, medical professionals insist that very soon pharmaceutical robots will lower the chances of error to near zero.

This would sharply contrast with today's standard procedure, in which drugs distributed within hospitals are directly given or administered to patients by highly trained human pharmacists or other medical professionals including nurses and doctors.

Shocking Development Stuns Industry

In perhaps the most stunning and emotionally shocking change, if engineers and scientists have their way, robotic devices will gradually replace all humans in the task of prescribing, preparing and distributing prescriptions within hospitals.

Although the overall planned transition is likely to change or evolve somewhat in unpredictable ways, here is the primary overall plan--as envisioned by many officials:

Pharmacy environment: Within the actual pharmacy, by the mid-2020s, moving mechanical machines or robotic devices will travel among shelves--collecting and measuring pharmaceuticals. The machines are programmed to perform these tasks with great efficiency, accurately completing the prescription orders as mandated by human physicians. Also, during the 2020s amid this initial transition, after collecting the right amount of drugs the machines will deliver the orders to "human pharmacists" inside those facilities. From that point, pharmacy or hospital personnel take the drugs to the assigned or designated locations within the facility. At those locations, human medical professionals administer the drugs to patients--similar to the process from the 2010s. Yet all this is set to change dramatically by the mid- to late-2020s. In the most stunning or seemingly unbelievable transition in hospital pharmacology, humans will either largely--or even fully--be eliminated from this drug issuing and distributing process. Remember, as previously mentioned, this is already happening at a handful of North American hospitals. Also, even more shockingly, if many robotics experts and medical facility administrators have their way, all prescriptions will eventually be issued by RoboDocs, rather than by human doctors. From today's perspective, such a transition might seem impossible, ludicrous and even unimaginable. Yet this fails to take away the fact that such a "takeover" by robots has been planned and envisioned by those creating such devices.

In-Hospital Distribution: With steadily increased efficiency, while also eliminating the need for certain employees, by the mid- to late-2020s, machines deliver the issued pharmaceuticals to patient rooms on a 24-hour basis. This will mark a significant change from just a decade earlier when many hospitals maintained in-hospital pharmacies that were opened and operating for a limited number of hours daily. By the mid- to late 2030s, robots--rather than humans--will deliver prescribed drugs to patient rooms, ICUs and other in-hospital treatment areas; this is the same aforementioned process already happening on a limited basis. The final phase of this transition will mark a significant change from the late 2020s. At the point where human doctors and nurses have largely been eliminated from the equation, machines will administer the drugs to patients; this process will range from installing IVs, to injections and administering pills on highly regimented, pre-set schedules.

Issuing prescriptions: As previously indicated, under some plans the actual prescriptions would be issued by robots or automated machines--rather than by human doctors. The "decision" by such a device is to be based on specific pre-set criteria, largely taking into account various factors including: the patient's vital signs; the diagnosis or underlying medical issue; the person's medical history; the effectiveness of drugs already given to the person; and the calculated probability of improving the patient's health. The robots' assigned or pre-programmed roles will be to eliminate adverse symptoms, and to enable the person to resume a "normal life."

Super-intelligence: According to scientists and electrical engineers, certain individual robots in the future will be hundreds of times "smarter" than average humans. Already well along in the planning and development stages, this roll-out of super-intelligence is scheduled to click into full gear on a massive scale throughout society from the mid-2020s to the mid-2030s. Essentially, the "brains" of an individual high-performance robot will be simultaneously connected to numerous supercomputers. Just as is the case today, each of these data systems is programmed with billions or even trillions of bits of information. When collectively functioning as a single unit, theoretically these devices have all "known human knowledge." These factors, in turn, serve as the supposed justification for allowing higher-level robots to make life-and-death decisions impacting human patients.

Chapter 6
Robotic Limbs

Besides machines that perform tasks in hospitals and clinics, by mid-2015 scientists had made huge advancements in developing "robotic limbs" for people.

The bulk of these significant developments resulted from research motivated by horrific injuries suffered by U.S. military personnel in Iraq and Afghanistan.

Thousands of soldiers lost some or all of their arms or legs; the wounds initially left many of these people unable to walk or to perform basic tasks.

At the start of these wars in early 2002, machines or prosthetic devices were relatively crude by today's standards.

Unsatisfied with those early techniques, electrical engineers engaged in a complex artificial-limb development and testing program. Thanks to these efforts, the latest updated devices sharply boost the patients' bodily motor skills.

Significant Developments Occurred

Many of the most advanced robotic limbs easily perform their required tasks. This factor, in turn, sharply improves the overall quality of life for each patient.

Among factors that make these high-performance machines efficient are:

Physical Integration: In many instances, certain brands of these robotic limbs are connected to the patient's brain functions. When all goes as planned, the person is able to easily command movements in artificial fingers, hands or feet--plus entire limbs.

Costs: Although per-unit costs typically reach many thousands of dollars, expenses are typically borne by the U.S. Veterans Administration.

Employment possibilities: Particularly among the users of these devices who have not been listed as "fully disabled," robotic limbs enable many of them to get jobs--often enhancing these patients' sense of self-worth.

The **"Relative Factor:"** Thanks to these improvements, relatives or care-givers of the injured often feel as if a significant burden has been lifted. In some instances, the artificial limbs sharply decrease any need for people other than the patient to assist in everyday lifestyle tasks, such as bathing or getting dressed.

Planned Improvements

Striving for more progress, the developers of robotic limbs hope to make additional significant improvements through the 2020s and beyond.

Many scientists and robotics professionals envision developing machines that will perform previously unheard-of abilities in aiding the sick or wounded. Among features:

Eyes: Artificial or high-functioning robotic eyes, used to replace such organs lost due to compat injuries, accidents or disease. These would be connected to integral optic nerves in the brain.

Ears: The loss of ear function due to horrific head injuries or extremely loud explosions would be corrected by implanting "robotic ears" into the head.

Joints: For many years, doctors have used fairly crude or rudimentary devices to replace damaged joints such as knees or hips. Yet if all goes as planned, such units in the future will be far more durable, reliable and natural than those of today. For instance, among patients undergoing hip replacements in the 2010s, operations were needed at least every 10 years for necessary replacements; the newer joints should last a lifetime.

Immunity: Foreign objects implanted inside or connecting into the body have historically caused potentially life-threatening immunity problems. Electrical engineers, working in conjunction with medical experts, plan to continue developing new technology to correct or eliminate this problem.

Wearable Robots

At the time of this book's initial publication, engineers had already made significant advancements in creating and building robotic parts that can be worn--even by healthy, non-disabled people.

Given the casual term of "wearable robots," depending on the specific type of device purchased, these machines were still under development on a wide-scale basis.

Under most of these plans, by the mid-2020s, initial models or brands of wearable robots will be available for purchase by patients and healthy consumers as well.

Some analysts projected extremely high consumer demand for these devices, although the effort had received little or no publicity during earlier development phases.

Amid the the initial transition stage, the companies creating wearable robotic applications had not revealed the projected retail prices.

Benefits of Wearable Machines

As previously mentioned, wearable robotic devices will offer or provide significant benefits to both healthy and disabled people using them. Among the most significant features:

Strength: Depending on how each specific mechanical unit is programmed, the devices could give real or perceived strength equal to--or far greater than--average humans.

Protection: Primarily in instances involving disabled people, wearable machines will provide a functional protective coating that prevents further injury.

Speed: High-functioning robotic legs will enable a person to run many times faster than even the speediest human. All this would be done using an internal robotics system that prevents damage to the person's flesh, organs and bones.

Power: Related to the "strength" factor mentioned earlier, some wearable units will give users tremendous physical power. Under tests in laboratory conditions, the strongest of these devices have enabled people to move, lift or push non-running cars.

Full-Body Robotic Devices

As outlandish as this might seem, some engineers also were developing robots that ultimately replace entire bodies--everything up to the head.

"This sounds stupid--unbelievable!" many people might proclaim upon first hearing this. "The notion of replacing an entire human body is pure nonsense."

Contrary to such statements, however, several researchers in Europe claimed they were well on their way to creating such functional devices. At least according to numerous predictions, by 2020 or perhaps much sooner, full-body units will be used and available at most major hospitals worldwide. Among features:

Human head: The heads of human beings would be attached to a robot. The device would be fully functional, mechanical from feet to neck.

Nerve systems: Using the latest super-technology, during the surgical phase nerves leading from the person's brain will be connected to the machine.

Bodily death: Everything from the neck down of the person's "flesh body" will die during the surgery. If the operation is successful, the person "technically and legally" will remain alive because brain function continues.

Move Over, Doctor Frankenstein

The notion of full-body robots seems like a warped, unbelievable plot from a modern Frankenstein movie.

Yet physicians and engineers working together in these combined efforts insist that society needs to prepare emotionally and financially for this critical transition. Several critical factors emerge on a moral and economic scale. Among primary issues.

Eternal life: People who can afford the full-body robots and eventually survive the procedure theoretically will have an opportunity to "live forever." This assumes, of course, that the scientists successfully develop methods to keep the brain alive.

Moral issues: Some people, particularly those ensconced into certain religions, might argue that "extending life this way is immoral--against God's wishes." Many of these protesters likely will include the same people who oppose abortion.

Ethical issues: Streams of people worldwide likely will complain that such a system would be "unfair," with only a limited number of individuals who can benefit--due to the extremely high cost.

Economic issues: The most heated controversies likely would center on the complaint, "Why should wealthy people be allowed to live forever or at least for hundreds of years, while the poor die?"

Cost factors: Another critical factor likely would involve who should pay for full-body robotic transplants and how. Whether insurance companies ever pay for such procedures remains unknown. Just as essential, U.S. politicians likely would have to decide whether to include such procedures under Medicare, Medicaid or the travesty of Obamacare.

Life-and-Death Decisions

By this juncture you surely must realize that the advent of medical robotics generates critical questions involving decisions on whether a person must live or die.

Authorities have faced similar questions for many generations, particularly each time significant advancements are made in medical care.

Every time we enjoy significant strides in medical technology, society finds itself faced with mind-boggling key issues that humanity never had to face before.

Prime examples from the past involved such landmark discoveries in the mid-20th Century as the cure for polio and life-saving penicillin.

Even so, huge segments of the global populations lacked access to these cures, during the initial decades after these landmark transitions. More than 60 years later, countless people worldwide still lack access to these "miracle cures."

Such instances help put the full-body robot issue into perspective, a realization that the expected controversy very likely will continue for many decades.

Download Your Personality

As if all these previously mentioned issues were not already enough to cause extensive worry, a new and related issue has emerged.

According to various news stories and press releases, scientists remain busy developing technology to "download your personality" into machines.

Even more disturbing, researchers have announced efforts to download information from your brain into computers. These factors, in turn, ignite many more issues and concerns. Among them:

Your soul: When downloading your personality and information from your brain into a computer, would technology be robbing you of your soul? Just as pressing, would, could or should a robot using your personality and personal data be "the real you?"

Death factor: Assuming that your entire body dies, but only after your personality and data have been downloaded--in a legal, moral and ethical sense would you still be considered "alive?"

Critical decisions: Particularly within the United States, politicians and the courts ultimately will need to make wide-scale and controversial decisions on these issues.

Condemned killers: Potentially bizarre and over-the-top situations might eventually occur, creating widespread disagreement throughout society. For instance, what if doctors downloaded the personality and brain of a condemned killer before authorities carry out the execution? Would officials then need to hunt down and destroy the "digitized remains" of the person?

48

Countless Issues Emerge

A seemingly endless stream of potential issues likely will emerge, due to the massive scope and impact of medical robotics.

Like this or not, as evidenced from the many examples already mentioned, the healthcare segment of robotics likely will generate intense debate and widespread controversy.

Among critical factors facing society:

Hospitals and health clinics: Administrators grapple with data and opinion surveys, to decide if cost factors and improved efficiency would justify such changes.

Patients and their families: These people weigh potential fear and worry with the notion that perhaps robotics and automated devices will improve their health.

Medical industry professionals: New medical school graduates, in the process of receiving their medical licenses, might discover "too late" that their hoped-for positions as physicians have been eliminated by robots.

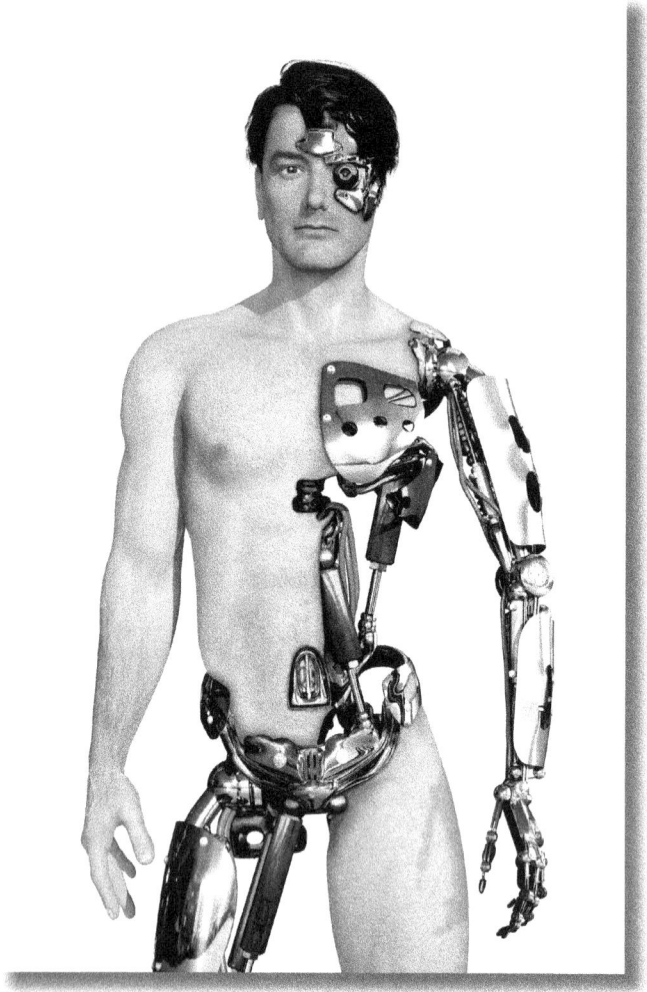

Chapter 7
Rehabilitation Robotics

Already rapidly growing at a super-charged pace by 2016, the burgeoning rehabilitation robotics industry was changing the entire health care process.

In some instances over hundreds or thousands of years, doctors and nurses have used rather crude devices in the patient rehabilitation process.

Through the pre-Iraq War era, typical rehabilitation tools ranged from non-moving rubber devices such as prosthetic arms to metal, hooked-shaped hands.

A wide range of ailments or injuries targeted for rehab range from the loss of limbs from war, disease or vehicular accidents, to helping seniors regain mobility after suffering falls.

Thanks to focus and determination by engineers, doctors and scientists, many of the basic mechanisms commonly used in this effort have evolved into robotics.

Specialized Functions Evolved

On a medical level, doctors and rehabilitation specialists developed this specialized robotics segment to enhance each patient's "sensorimotor functions."

This term designates the function and effectiveness of a person's ability to effectively move everything from hands, legs and toes, to arms and feet.

In optimal and high-performing rehab facilities, the human rehab professionals now using robotic devices strive to maximize the effectiveness of two primary regimens:

Therapeutic Training: These entail "control strategies for robotic movement training after injury," according to a June 2009 article in the "Journal of NeuroEngineering and Rehabilitation."

Sensorimotor Performance: Scientists study the effectiveness of robots to enhance or improve upper limb function after strokes, according to a November 2012 article in the

"American Journal of Physical Medicine & Rehabilitation."

Rehab experts use the updated technology as higher functioning therapy aids, rather using them as merely "assistive devices."

For the most part, according to at least some published reports, patients generally tolerate robotic therapies. Some healthcare professionals consider robots as an "effective adjunct" for improving a patient's motor skills--especially after strokes.

Biomedical Engineering

Like many other forms of medical robots, the machines used for rehabilitation are within the burgeoning "biomedical engineering" process that assists doctors and patients.

This term designates the ongoing effort to meld the realms of medicine and engineering, according to a 2012 publication, "Introduction to Biomedical Engineering," by John Denis Enderle and Joseph D. Bronzino.

Within the overall biomedical engineering process, experts in medicine and engineering work together; they strive to advance or significantly improve health care.

Through each step in the machine development and creation process, biomedical engineers strive to sharply improve three essential processes:

Diagnosis: Enhancing and improving robots and technical equipment used to determine the cause, source and level of the patient's illness or medical condition.

Monitoring: Maximizing the effectiveness of devices that continually check the patient's health, everything from basic vital signs to muscle function.

Therapy: Rehabilitation processes that generally occur on regimented, pre-set schedules designed to enhance health while improving the patient's mobility.

Improving Overall Rehabilitation

The joint effort by healthcare professionals and mechanical

engineers began accelerating in 1989, the inaugural year of the International Conference on Rehabilitation Robotics.

Thanks to this important organization, these industry experts meet every two years to share vital information and bolster their combined effort.

They have steadily made significant strides at improving the overall rehab industry, maximizing positive results from therapy regimens--as engineers continually develop new robots.

Sadly, however, this combined effort has received scant attention in the mainstream media, even though such landmark developments are steadily beging made.

As a result, most people remain unaware that these machines exist, until they or their relatives need to undergo robot-assisted rehab regimens.

Basic Types of Rehab Robots
On a wide-scale basis, the overall robotics industry has had two basic types of machines:

Mechanical: These devices perform repetitive pre-programmed functions, movements that never or rarely vary to any significant degree.

High-functioning: These have a broader range of potential movements and many more functions, in some instances "thinking" or regulated by computer "brains."

Although rare exceptions have occurred, the vast majority of rehab robots used through the first decade of the 21st Century were low-function mechanical machines.

Thanks to significant advancements in biomedical engineering, the rehab industry is poised for significant enhancements and improvements through the 2030s and beyond.

Early Prototypes Electrified the Industry
Within several years after the Conference on Rehabilitation Robotics began, medical and engineering experts introduced significant improvements in rehabilitation.

Initial strides kicked into gear during the early to mid-1990s, when these professionals introduced robots specialized in addressing neurological disorders.

According to various published reports, certain robots that specialize in this aspect of the rehabilitation industry have been able to:

Sensing: Particularly among patients suffering nervous system disorders, the machines enable the person to recognize objects by touching them.

Assisting: Robots help or assist individual patients, enabling the people to balance or stand, and in some instances to enhance the person's "gait"--the natural and effective pattern of limb movements.

Partly due to the complexity of these necessary tasks, developing effective rehabilitation robots has been challenging. Luckily, however, this has been far from impossible thanks to steadily improving technology.

Overcoming Challenges

Potentially significant obstacles have posed challenges for the developers of these machines. The research and robot-creation process involves far more than merely designing and building rehab machines on a quick and massive scale.

Instead, engineers with the continual assistance of medical experts have had to identify, map out and mimic the bodily movements and reactions of "real-live humans."

At face value this overall task might seem easy. Yet the process has been time-consuming and arduous, primarily because humans are highly complex creatures.

To make this happen, for many years scientists systematically studied human movements in laboratories, using digital technology to record every subtle movement.

As if this overall challenge were not already enough, researchers then had to development precise new robotic mechanical systems that precisely mimic the unique way that humans move their limbs and entire bodies.

The Blend Between Humans and Robots

As you will soon discover in far more detail in subsequent chapters, the goal of making machines like--or even better than--humans is the primary challenge facing engineers.

Within rehabilitation, this blending of human and machine has emerged as equal to--or even more essential than--most other specialized segments of the robotics industry.

As an overall sector, rehab robots have unique attributes that in many instances are vastly different from machines serving any other business or segment of society:

Disabled: Unlike other robots, these machines are designed to work specifically with disabled people--who each have unique challenges that healthy people lack.

Safety: Like some specific robots designed for other businesses, the rehab devices must react fast if something goes wrong during a rehabilitation session.

Stupendous Results

Today's rehab robots have won rave reviews for their verified ability to assist and to improve the health of patients.

Such positive commentaries likely will continue at an increasing pace, particularly as improved or updated robot models enter the marketplace.

Even before that expected transition, most or all rehabilitation medical facilities already offer some form of robotic device patients.

Meantime, is there a possiblity that some or even all human employees at rehab facilities will lose their jobs--their tasks taken over by specialized robots?

The answer seems difficult to pinpoint. However, if this sector eventually mirrors most robotics advancements, some people at those facilities probably will lose their jobs--perhaps one or two decades from now.

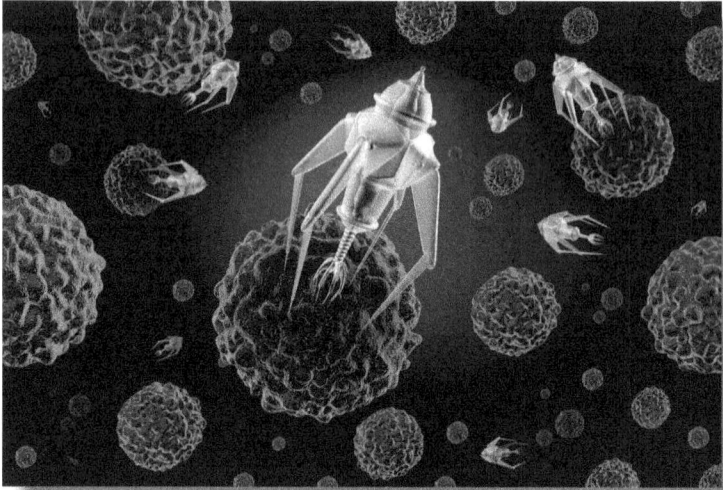

Chapter 8
Biomedical Engineering and Nanotechnology

The previously mentioned "biomedical engineering process" plays an increasingly critical role in almost every aspect of ongoing and vital developments in medical technology--one of which is robotics.

Remember that this process, sometimes called "BME," blends biology and medicine with basic engineering principles. Working closely with doctors and biologists, engineers design devices essential to improving health care.

While the science of robotics plays an increasingly vital role in this wide-scale process, a variety of other disciplines become "inter-related."

This means that various scientific realms require their own advancements or discoveries in order to eventually generate improvements in another realm--such as robotics.

For instance, thanks to biological advancements in brain research engineers have been able to design and build the aforementioned machines that download personalities and data.

Atom-sized Robots

As part of the science and study called "nanotechnology," engineers and biologists have worked together to build atom-sized robots. The human scientists create these miniscule devices by mixing specific chemicals, thereby forming tiny movements controlled by magnetic forces.

As bizarre and strange as this might seem, this rapidly growing field has steadily become increasingly important in medicine and basic health care.

In fact, nano-robots have quickly become so vital to medicine that you will be learning far more about this feature in a subsequent chapter.

The development of these super-miniaturized devices became possible largely as the result of advancements in the biological research into the human genome.

Various fields of science have rapidly blended together in this overall process since 1990, when researchers made significant discoveries in biology and engineering.

Medicine's Tiny Allies

As of 2016, medical professionals already were using or planning to implement advancements in nanotechnology for the treatment of human patients. Amid these efforts in initial stages, scientists were beginning:

Heart treatment: Using the miniature robots, roughly the size as blood cells, to clean or remove life-threatening plaque from arterial walls.

Cancer: Undergoing studies and tests designed to enable atom-sized robots to deliver bee venom to cancer cells, eventually killing those invaders.

Infections: Developing nano-robots to assist the body's natural white blood cells in battling infections and biological invaders.

Although receiving relatively little publicity in the mainstream media, these mini-scale medical advancements were progressing at a steady pace.

Positive Developments Expected

Many medical and engineering experts hope to drastically improve health care in steadily improved phases through the 2030s, thanks largely to nanotechnology.

Yet none of this will happen unless researchers are able to unlock more biological "secrets," specifically the internal makeup of all cells in the human body.

With dogged persistence, and following a careful plan, during the next few decades experts hope to use nano-robots to control many ailments. Among them:

Diabetes: Regulating blood sugars to optimal levels for good health.

Alzheimer's: Cleaning or removing substances that degrade cognitive ability.

Diagnosis: Briefly touring the entire body to find and target health problems.

For now, many of these goals are merely part of a "pie-in-the-sky" wish list. But scientists insist these objectives are well within the realm of possibility.

"Virgin" Technology

As compared to most scientific endeavors, biomedical engineering has only recently evolved into its own category or field of study.

Far than merely tiny robots, this effort involves or assists in monitoring, diagnosis and therapy, according to a 2012 book, "Introduction to Biomedical Engineering," by John Denis Enderle and Joseph D. Bronzino.

Besides the previously mentioned biomedical prostheses, some that include robotic attributes, the miniature devices or machines--already in service or under development--range from micro-implants to clinical equipment.

Besides "therapeutic biologicals" and pharmaceutical drugs, the many other devices or substances generated by biomedical engineering include non-robotic machines; these include EEGs and MRIs.

Among the most widely known to the general public are non-invasive ultrasound devices that scan internal organs like the bladder, uterus, kidneys and prostate.

Many Specialties Involved

As briefly mentioned earlier, the overall biomedical engineering sector involves many subsets or fields of study. Each vital to the treatment, diagnosis and monitoring of specific diseases or adverse medical conditions, these include:

Tissue engineering: This segment of biotechnology concentrates on bodily tissues, usually individual organs. A primary goal is to use biological materials to re-create or regrow vital regions of the body. Robotics eventually might play a significant role in this effort.

Genetic engineering: Made possible by significant discoveries in genetics, this effort strives to manipulate or modify a person's DNA in order to eradicate or prevent ailments. Robotics might eventually play a role in diagnosis or changing the DNA.

Neural engineering: Much more work is needed in this highly complex realm that involves the body's nervous system. Robotics devices or extremely small machines might eventually play a primary role in diagnosis, repair or nerve replacement.

Pharmaceutical engineering: As the name implies, this involves the designing and creation of drugs. Eventually, nano-robots might play a role in diagnosis, data collection, or perhaps even in the aforementioned drug manufacturing process.

Giant Strides Expected

On a broad scale, giant strides can be expected as biomedical engineering improves and creates new technologies well into the 2030s and beyond.

Precisely how much of a role robotics will play a role in these specific efforts remains unknown. Yet if past and present advancements are any indication, in all likelihood various kinds of robots will play essential roles.

"The greatest discoveries and uses for robots for medical uses are still on the horizon," I tell any patient who might inquire. "Particularly among patients who are young today, medical robots are likely to change their lives or even bring good health."

Many people fail to realize this, but biomedical engineering already has drastically improved health care since 1990. As a result, many types of devices have been introduced into medical treatment, technology that most consumers "take for granted."

The steadily growing list of these devices, many built using automated "non-thinking" robots include: dental implants; pacemakers; kidney dialysis machines; artificial organs; infusion pumps; heart-lung machines; facial prosthetics; ocular prosthetics; corrective lenses; and many other devices, too numerous to list in full.

Understand "Stereolithography"

The system-wide advancements and growth of biomedical engineering has generated an additional scientific system called "stereolithography."

In basic terms, this involves "medical modeling" or using the known characteristics of biological substances, and mapping out and creating physical objects.

To make this happen, ultimately creating the building blocks for generating objects such as tissue, scientists must map biological characteristics on an atomic level.

Once again, robotics and nanotechnology are likely to play increasingly crucial roles as this integral aspect or subset of health care.

Like "Shooting for the Moon."

In a sense, the overall biomedical engineering effort of today is the equivalent of striving to land on the moon back in the 1960s, except for one major difference.

The moon-landing effort received extensive media publicity during that decade, while the average person today knows little or nothing about medical robotics.

The public's support for space exploration swelled after President John F. Kennedy vowed to have the USA land on the moon before the end of that decade. Later, upon NASA's initial landing of men on the moon in July 1969--nearly six years after an assassin killed Kennedy, the public across America and worldwide celebrated that remarkable achievement.

By comparison, the vast majority of people today lack any

hint of the milestone advances in robotics and that transition's potentially positive impact on health care. So at least for now the public lacks any opportunity to cheer about advances in medical robotics, while mesmerized by compelling images of medical robots on their TVs.

When initially walking on the moon, the late astronaut Neil Armstrong famously said, "One small step for man; one giant leap for mankind."

In a sharp contrast, the steady rollout of robots into medicine during the next few decades might emerge as equally important to humanity, yet without public celebrations.

Clinical Engineering

The eventual success or failure of the medical robots will hinge on "clinical engineering," a relatively new branch within biomedical engineering.

On both a scientific and business level, clinical engineering involves the process and implementation of new medical technology and equipment into hospitals and clinics.

Combining the realms of biology and engineering, people involved in this branch hold a high-degree of responsibility for performing numerous tasks. Those include:

Training and supervising: Carefully chosen clinical engineers that teach medical personnel how to use or implement new high-tech equipment or services.

Requirements: Work in conjunction with auditors, inspectors and government regulators; bureaucrats at various federal agencies must approve any new technology before that specific method or system can be used in medical facilities.

Consultation: Especially during periods where certain technologies are "all-new" to the healthcare industry, give advice to doctors and hospital administrators.

Production: Give much-needed advice to manufactures of medical devices, even when producers strive to integrate prospective design improvements. Some of these vital communications feature comments from doctors who describe their clinical experiences with a specific device; the physicians and engineers give their suggestions on how to improve the efficiency of medical tools.

Robotics Enters the "Grand Scheme of Things"

All current and future medical robots must first be thoroughly reviewed and approved by authorities before doctors and hospitals use them.

According to some published reports, most clinical engineers focus primarily on the incremental or regular upgrading of products already used by hospitals and doctors.

Less of these professionals' time, resources and personal energy reportedly goes toward revolutionary new technology and developments such as medical robots.

However, during the five-year period before this book's publication, scientists seemed eager to intensify their efforts to create new innovations

The ultimate decisions on whether to actively pursue medical robotics innovation will rest with the consumer marketplace--the real or perceived demand from the general public. Basic decisions will hinge on profit potential; this involves calculating whether research and developmenet efforts would ultimately "pay for themselves" by creating income-generating technology.

Extensive Employee Requirements

As demand swells for people with extensive mathematical and medical skills, several universitities have started offering courses that lead to degrees in Bachelor of Science Biomedical Engineering.

The students who earn good grades position themselves for a significantly higher probability of high-paying robotics-related jobs, especially developing machines for health care. Some students land these lucrative jobs a year or two before graduation.

Successful candidates have a keen understanding of both engineering and biology. This unique and specialized knowledge enables them to consider and blend critical aspects of these two fields when envisioning, designing and creating medical devices.

Profit potential increases among bioengineering firms that successfully recruit the most talented and qualified recent graduates who specialize in robotics.

A steadily growing number of universities are becoming accredited by the Accreditation Board for Engineering and Technology, Inc., often called "ABET." According to this non-governmental organization, its primary function involves accrediting post-secondary education programs or institutions; these specialize in engineering technology, applied science, engineering and computing.

According to a report issued in early 2012 by ABET, the organization had accredited more than 3,200 programs at 670 colleges and universities in 23 countries.

An "occupational handbook" issued for 2014-2015 by the U.S. Bureau of Labor Statistics confirmed that such graduates were in high demand. Government statisticians estimated that the number of biomedical engineers would grow 27 percent by 2022.

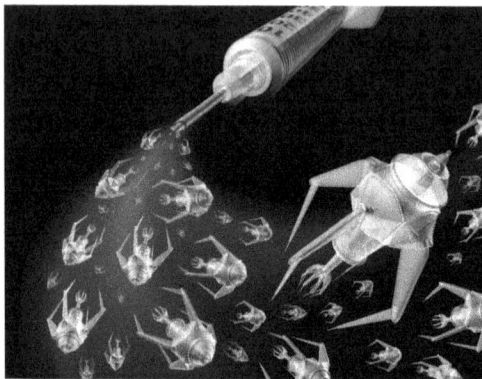

Chapter 9
Microscopic-sized Robots

Briefly mentioned earlier, amazingly in recent years scientists have been able to envision and to create robots as small as atoms.

On a universal measuring scale typically used by scientists these manmade devices can be as small as one "nanometre." To put this in perspective, that's one billionth of a meter; the term nanometre is sometimes used to express measurements on an atomic scale.

But why do some doctors want such miniature machines?

The answers rest in fairly new and rapidly emerging field of scientific research and study called "nanorobotics."

These advancements have been verified by numerous organizations and public reports, including: the National Council on Disability; scientific research papers; and the Tennessee-based Office of Scientific and Technical Information.

Steady Advancements

Although most advancements in nanorobotics are still in the research and development phase, scientists already have been able to test new devices that include:

Nanomotors: These molecular-sized devices convert energy into movement. If research and technological advancements continue as expected, these devices will be able to interact with the body's essential motor proteins found within living cells. Ideally, nanomotors will be able to transport substances such as medication into living cells. According to a 2004 research report in the "Journal of American Chemistry," scientists at Penn State University created "catalytic nanowire motors" that are autonomously able to propel themselves thanks to the presence of a hydrogen peroxide fuel.

Molecular Machines: Sometimes called "nanomachines,"

these microscopic devices use a specific stimuli to produce quasi-mechanical movements, according to a 2001 report by the "Accounts of Chemical Research," a peer-review scientific journal--published by the American Chemical Society. Scientists classify two categories of molecular machines, "synthetic" and "biological."

A primary goal of these atomic-size devices is to build what researchers call "molecular assemblers."

American engineer K. Eric Drexler, who earned his doctoral theses at the Massachusetts Institute of Technology, has said that these proposed devices are "able to guide chemical reactions by positioning reactive molecules with atomic precision."

The Association of American Publishers gave its 1992 Best Computer Science Book Award to Drexler for "Nanosystems: Molecular Machinery Manufacturing and Computation." Thanks to groundbreaking work by Drexler and other scientists, starting in 2007 the British Engineering and Physical Sciences Council started funding efforts to create ribosome-like molecular assemblers. In basic terms, a "ribosome" is a complex living molecular machine naturally found within cells used to transport proteins.

If successful as many scientists predict, nanorobotics eventually will be able to interact with, change or regulate the human body's otherwise natural process of "biological protein synthesis." This involves the regulation of amino acids and proteins, all essential to good health.

Under the leadership of the Battelle Memorial Institute, scientists at various research facilities affiliated with U.S. National Laboratories keep busy exploring how to build and manage nanorobots--using atomically precise technologies.

Advancements Accelerate

The level of optimism increased among scientists after they performed tests during early phases in the development of nanorobots.

According to various published reports, researchers managed to develop and monitor sensors as small as 1.5 nanometers wide.

These developments motivated doctors, biologists and researchers to launch another all-new field of study called "nanomedicine." This growing branch of the overall healthcare industry conducts what the term implies, medicine on an atomic scale.

Thanks to these efforts, the healthcare industry in recent years has for the first time been able to use machines to monitor and manipulate living cells.

Amazingly, only a small percentage of people have ever heard of miniature robots, although these steadily emerging medical advancements continue to acceelrate.

Entering a New Realm

Perhaps most people "remain clueless" about these significant discoveries because the majority of us throughout society pay little attention to such complex details.

Over the course of the next several years, however, chances seem strong that these advancements will become popular, particularly when and if nanorobots eventually regulate or even kill cancer as some scientists hope.

For this to happen, intense research and new technologies will be needed from the emerging sub-fields and medical applications of nanomedicine. Among them are:

Nanomaterials: Manmade and natural objects measured in nanometers or even small portions of nanometers.

Biological devices: Commonly called "BioBricks," these structures are the basic materials used in assembling and designing biological circuits.

If research and development goes as planned, scientists will be able to incorporate or introduce biological devices into living cells. According to a March 2014 article in the "Journal of

Biological Engineering," and other reports, BioBricks eventually will be used in constructing new biological systems within such cells; targeted living substances at the cellular level include Escherichia coli, commonly found in the intestines of warm-blooded organisms. Although mostly harmless, some strains cause food poisioning.

Nanoelectronic Biosensors: These devices within the field of nanotechnology use electronic components; these manmade objects cause inter-atomic interactions so small that scientists seem to agree much more study is needed. The vast majority of these biosensors are used by--or planned for--a wide varity of non-medical uses. These range from computers and memory storage to on-screen displays, radios and energy production. At least one medical field is likely to benefit, primarily diagnostics. According to a 2008 article in "Medical Product Manufacturing News," scientists are interested in using nanoelectronic biosensors in developing and using a still-to-be-developed process using nanosensors in real-time diagnostics; these will effectively monitor concentrations of biomolecules.

Molecular Nanotechnology: This emerging field involves the building of complex atomic structures. To do this, scientists hope to use a chemical syntheses process that--if effective--would drive certain "reactive molecules" to specific molecular sites. This would be achieved by generating a series of complex chemical reactions.

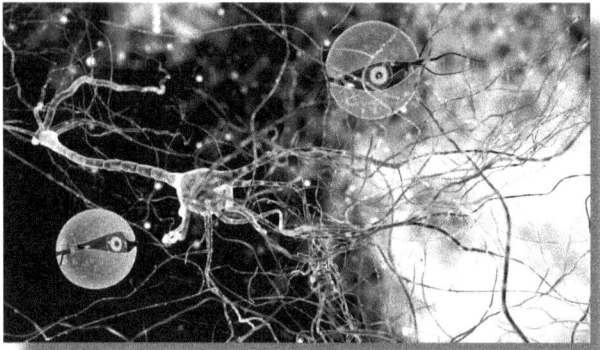

Chapter 10
Nanorobots Battle Disease

The many potential benefits of cell- or atomic-sized robots are already viewed as the "cure of the future" by many medical industry professionals and busines analysts.

As far back as September 2009, a theoretical lifetime in the rapid advancement of medical technology, the "Wall Street Journal" noted that nanorobots would eventually play a significant role in fighting cancer.

Briefly mentioned earlier, the bee-venom strategy of fighting the disease with nanorobots as delivery mechanisms finally got considered.

Prior to that, for many decades or even centuries societies worldwide had viewed that many various forms of venom as potential remedies for eradicating the disease.

Yet until recently scientists had a major problem in delivering the venom to healthy cells. Without going straight to the cancer, the venom would kill or decimate otherwise healthy, necessary and beneficial cells including nerves.

Such potential dangers are on the verge of getting blocked or eliminated, but only if scientists can build or "train" nanorobots to effectively deliver venom to specific locations inside the diseased cells.

Introducing "Nanobees"
The higly specialized venom-delivering miniature robots, some a size equal to human cells, are called "nanobees." This research is already at a relatively early stage; if all goes as hoped the devices theoretically could start working full-scale by 2025.

In May 2015, the "Madcast Gaming" news site quoted doctors and scientists who predicted that nanobees could emerge as a "conventional" therapy in treating cancer. Research also indicated the technique effectively killed pre-cancerous cells.

A specialist in nanomedicine from Washington University in Saint Louis, Professor Samuel Wickline, told the publication that the nanobees essentially seem to "fly" in via the blood stream, "land on the surface of cells and deposit their poisonous cargo."

Based on ongoing research, this unique and highly specialized delivery system likely will emerge as so popular that it might replace conventional oncology therapy, according to a report published by the "Journal of Clinical Investigation."

Early Results Proved Promising

According to the "Madcast" article, research scientists used two groups of mice suffering from cancerous tumors--melanoma, and human breast cancer that had been injected.

"After four to five injections of the nanobees, the breast cancer tumors were 25 percent smaller, and the melanoma tumors were 88 percent smaller," when compared to untreated mice, the article said.

Government agencies had given approval for those initial tests. Researchers told journalists they were hopeful that during 2016 they would be able to use nanobees in test trials on human cancer patients.

The researchers predicted several potential benefits, if the tests proved that nanobees are beneficial:

Health issues: Fewer adverse side effects than conventional cancer treatment.

Effectiveness: Better results than conventional chemotherapy.

Dosage levels: Some oncologists give patients the "highest tolerable" dosage levels of chemotherapy, which destroy healthy cells--potentially leading to extremely adverse symptoms or even death. By contrast, when using nanobees, doctors would deliver doses in much smaller amounts because the devices only target diseased cells.

Extreme Caution Recommended

As one of only a handful of licensed integrative medical oncologists practicing in the United States, I would advise doctors and researchers from becoming overly optimistic about the apparent ability of nanobees to deliver venom in fighting cancer in humans.

You see, the venom from bees, snakes and other animals is a natural substance. By law, pharmaceutical companies cannot patent substances found in nature.

Like this or not, the situation poses a huge potential roadblock for such entrepreneurial efforts--even if effective and no matter how "well-intentioned."

The heart of this problem rests with the disturbing fact that drug companies care more about making profit for themselves-- than they do for using natural substances to save people.

Tragically, as fully chronicled in many of my other publications, the drug companies--nicknamed BigPharma-- play a powerful role in controlling the U.S. medical industry. And disturbingly, the pharmaceutical industry has tremendous political power, particularly regarding the medical review process conducted by federal bureaucrats. As a result, BigPharma is likely to use influencde the decisions made by bureaucrats who must consider whether to approve the devices.

Greed Endangers Consumers

All this comes down to the "Almighty Dollar," with BigPharma placing profit as a far higher prioritiy than actually saving people's lives.

The drug companies generate many billions of dollars yearly making and distributing chemo products that sicken or even kill cancer patients.

If the past is any indication of future performance, BigPharma will work diligently to prevent nanobees from becoming a standard cancer treatment. Otherwise, the drug companies would lose their lucrative, non-stop "Big Cash

Machine"--the deadly chemo drugs.

Using its typical "weaponry" in striving to block and disallow effective natural substances, BigPharma has the infrastructure to engage in a "political juggernaut."

Campaign contributions: Politicians nationwide, particularly those in Congress, receive many millions of dollars in campaign contributions from BigPharma. As a so-called payback, lawmakers fight against natural remedies that would lower drug company profits--while lowering consumer costs and significanlty improving health care.

Bureaucracy: Federal agencies that regulate and monitor the healthcare industry are filled with employees closely allied to BigPharma. Many of these bureaucrats once worked for major drug companies. The same people manage and set policy at agencies like the federal Food and Drug Administration (FDA) and the National Institutes of Health (NIH.)

Crony decisions: Kowtowing to the desires or demands of BigPharma, the federal bureaucrats almost always invariably deny applications for unique and effective technologies for delivering natural medicines into the body.

Will Government Corruption Stall Medical Robotics?

These disturbing factors bring forth an obvious question that deserves much further detail and analysis: "Will mainstream doctors and BigPharma fight against any effort to legalize highly advanced, autonomous and effective medical robots.

As you likely very well imagine from the many aforementioned examples, drug companies and mainstream allopathic physicians likely will do whatever is legally necessary to protect their Giant Cash Cow.

But would mainstream doctors launch such political battles, even if doing so meant preventing the public from getting significant improvements in health care?

Only "time will tell," partly because many of these proposed drastic changes likely would surprise many mainstream doctors; remember that as previously stated, many of them remain unaware of these advancements.

Consider My Unique Perspective

Although you might not have heard my name until now, several people have called me a "rock star within the medical industry."

At many of these gatherings that I attend or make speeches, many doctors greet me with applause and standing ovations.

Some medical professionals consider me as a visionary at spotting milestone trends, often before the transitions occur throughout the healthcare industry.

Envision the sense of disgust federal bureaucrats felt, knowing that my cancer treatment methods rely primarily on natural substances--rather than dangerous drugs.

Consumers deem my protocol as significant; at the back of this book, I have included a bonus section detailing my clinic's effective and natural cancer treatments.

Put the Situation into Perspective

Assuming that nanobees eventually get governmental approval, to put the overall situation into perspective, consider the following factors:

Homeopathic physicians: The upgraded system likely would benefit the livelihood of homeopaths who administer natural medicine.

Cancer patients: Assuming that nanobees become effective and win approval from bureaucrats, people suffering from cancer, particularly at advanced Stage IV levels, probably would never have to endure potentially fatal chemotherapy.

Under such a landmark transition, BigPharma and mainstream allopathic physicians would suffer a much-deserved severe economic setback.

Add to this the fact that only a handful of clinics including mine could administer nanobees, and then the political situation would grow into a proverbial powder keg.

As a result, a political firestorm is on the verge of erupting, amid the planned or potential wide-scale rollout of medical robots throughout the healthcare industry.

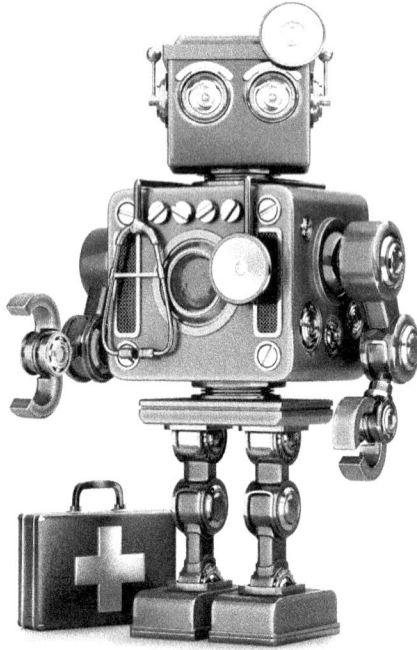

"RoboDocs"

Chapter 11
Political War Looms

At least for now, little mention seems to exist in the mainstream media and medical reports regarding how doctors, hospitals and BigPharma will react to what I call "The Rise of the Medical Robots."

From my perspective, based on known and published facts about the rapid development of such devices, a full-scale political war looms in the near future.

Yet this will be unlike standard politial battles or ideologies that are discussed in "open public forms," such as debates or mainstream news articles.

Instead, I envision an internal "cold war" throughout the medical industry and related bureaucracies--with little mention in the overly liberal, corrupt and inept mainstream media.

If that happens, consumers and patients would get locked out of the discussion and decision process. This seems likely, largely because today's average consumer lacks any hint that these technologies are being fine-tuned worldwide.

Consider Internal Business Factors

With "profit" and "greed" serving as proverbial the king and queen, those involved in the medical industry will make key decisions involving healthcare robots. Among these officials:

Hospitals: Expect administrators to carefully study the "bottom-line," such as whether eliminating human nurses and pharmacists will substantially boost profit.

BigPharma: With greed as its primary motivation, the drug industry likely will only push for robotics poised to increase that business sector's annual revenue.

Doctors: Although backed by powerful organizations such as the American Medical Association, human physicians might find themselves "in a pinch." Some hospitals and clinics might consider human doctors as expendable, particularly if engineers generate advanced "RoboDocs" just as skilled or better than the doctors.

Medical Schools: Some analysts have predicted that a huge percentage of all universities will close; this would happen partly for economic reasons, and also because robots and automated systems will eventually fill all primary jobs. Some robotics and business experts predict this transition will span the full scale of human knowledge and industry. As that transition occurs, people supposedly will have less motivation to seek benefits from higher education. Even so, when and if this transition begins, people with extensive medical knowledge initially will be needed--at least temporarily--in designing, creating and building fully functional "RoboDocs."

The "Unseen War."

From my view, following intense fact-finding and analysis by my research team, the reasons and impacts of this "power grab" will be vast and varied:

Universal change: The gradual but steadily increasing rollout of robots, permeating every business sector throughout society and in most cultures, will become common-place and routine in the minds of consumers. Largely as a result, as robotics enter various social systems and businesses, in the minds of many people medical machines will be "just another piece of an increasingly confusing puzzle"--which continually change everyone's life.

Public acceptance: If this massive rollout of robots occurs as analysts predict, consumers everywhere will feel increasingly dependant on the machines. Similar to the way most people feel as if they cannot live without the Internet, huge sections of society likely will demand more effective automated systems such as robotics in medicine--even in instances where such systems do not yet exist.

Inter-connected systems: If some business analysts who carefully study the advant of robotics are to be believed, machines and software-based automated systems will drastically change the everyday routines of most people. The involvement of robots in everything from transportation to food distrubtion will require people to modify their everyday activities.

Industrialized nations: The most evident revolutionary changes initially will impact industrialized nations where businesses deem robots as essential. This should happen within regions with the greatest profit potential.

Understand the "Battle Zones"

Unlike standard wars between armies that have deadly weapons, the behind-the-scenes battles over dominance in medical robots will lack clearly defined battlefronts. The "players" in this unpublicized cold war will have three objectives:

Money: The institutions, companies or individuals that "win" control or rights to build, maintain and control robots in one or more sectors of the healthcare industry will benefit the most; successful participants will position themselves for tremendous long-term profits. Remember that in the United States alone, medicine and health care is a multi-trillion-dollar industry. So, the "prize" is huge, a primary reason why this clandestine race is already well underway.

Power: Besides just money, those controlling or profiting from medical robotics will have tremendous clout. Particularly as consumers feel increasingly dependent on these devices, the robotics businesses and institutions likely will benefit financially-- thanks to a built-in monopoly protecting their positions.

Control: Related to power, any company or person with essential healthcare industry robotics patents likely will control all current and future activities within that business sector. Potential competitors striving to break these monopolies likely would lack the substantial funds needed to win the necessary government approval.

Identify the Likely Players

With literally trillions of dollars on the line, streams of medical businesses, institutions and healthcare professionals will engage in this internal power struggle.

In keeping with basic human nature, to varying degrees these "combatants" can be expected to zip into a "self-preservation mode."

This is the nature of almost all individuals, companies, institutions and organizations. Thus, we should expect an increasingly intense politial power play in Congress, in government bureaucracies and within business.

"Stay out of my territory," each participant would proclaim, without necessarily using such specific words. "The current rules are set in my favor, or--if that is not the case--I have allies that will make the crucial decisions on whether to accept or reject specific types of medical robots."

Remember, as previously stated, these powerful decision makers will not necessarily make the public's health and welfare their top priority--concentrating instead on maximizing profit.

Internal Struggles Commence

Predicting the short- and long-term outlook in this medical robotics power-play would be tantamount to trying to forecast the outcome of a pro football game many months beforehand. Nevertheless, the biggest probable players and their "game plans" seem obvious:

American Medical Association: Now more than 165 years old, and with at least 217,000 members, this mega-powerful organization is comprised of mainstream allopathic physicians, and even medical students. Some medical industry analysts believe that the association has close ties and a strong alliance with BigPharma. Some observers insist that this is largely why the mandatory patient treatment protocol regulating mainstream doctors requires them to prescribe extremely dangerous or even addictive drugs for specific medical conditions. According to "Our Corrupt

Politics ~ It's Not All Money," a 2012 book by Ezra Klein, the AMA has among the most powerful political lobbying budgets among any organization in the United States. This gives the association tremendous power in striving to control virtually all aspects of medicine. These factors enable the organization to play an integral role in controlling and regulating itself, particularly the actions or inactions of its members. With equal clout, some observers believe, the AMA also has the ability to prohibit certain substances or to prohibit certain behaviors by licensed or unlicensed people who provide medical services. Cognizant of the AMA's formidable power, an obvious question comes to mind: "While playing a signifant role in regulating its own industry, why and how would this organization ever allow 'mere robots' to serve as doctors?" Obviously, our world has always been an imperfect place. In theory the AMA should make the most ideal decisions, with all of its decisions and policies aggressively striving to enhance health care. Yet sadly, at least from the view of some critics, this organization has recklessly encouraged federal agencies to allow mega-pharmaceutical companies and doctors to produce or prescribe extremely dangerous drugs; many of these pharmaceuticals might cause a patient far more harm than good, often without specifically addressing the underlying medical condition. With a track record like this, from my view the precise way that the AMA will react to the introduction of medical robots is hard to predict. In all likelihood, when required approvals involve robotics, the organization's ultimate efforts will hinge on one primary factor--money. This generates an obvious question, "Who will benefit financially?" Yes, the build-up of "how to share the revenue pie" likely will emerge as a pivotal motivation. Despite its enormous political clout, the AMA has "lost" several political battles within the past century. Some of the most widely known failures were: the association's violation of the Sherman Antitrust Act, a decision affirmed by the U.S. Supreme Court; and the failure of the AMA's intense 1950s and 1960s campaign to block the creation of Medicare. Considering this imperfect track record, some observers might consider any attempt by the AMA to block the rollout of full-scale "robot doctors" as having an uncertain outcome.

BigPharma: Although often called by the nickname "BigPharma," this massive business sector is also occasionally labeled with the generic term: "pharmaceutical industry." According to several medical reports, by 2011 BigPharma's combined annual international revenues were just short of $1 trillion. Largely comprised of giant publicly traded companies, the firms produce, distribute and sell virtually all types of manmade drugs. These span a wide variety of pharmaceuticals, ranging from anti-inflammatories to highly addictive or even deadly painkillers. Although BigPharma and the AMA are not formally or directly affiliated, these separate organizations seem to work hand-in-hand--at least from the perspective of some critics. Like the AMA, BigPharma strives to protect its own interests. Ultimately, in most cases this strategy involves enacting legislation or bureaucratic rules requiring that doctors prescribe certain types of drugs for specific medical conditions. Also, like the AMA, BigPharma possesses substantial political power. Among key factors: thousands of drug industry lobbyists live in the Washington, D.C., area, developing close ties to Congress; the industry gives substantial campaign donations to politicians; the drug companies have close allies in federal agencies like the Food & Drug Administration (AMA); and en tandem with the medical association, the drug firms encourage instruction at medical schools that stresses the need to prescribe manmade drugs rather than natural substances for most ailments. From my view, consumers should expect BigPharma to fight any medical robotics system that might decrease that industry's revenues. Yet like the AMA, despite its own formidable clout and financial resources, BigPharma has failed to succeed in all of its political efforts. The most notable "loss" in this regard has been the steady increase in states that allow the use of medical marijuana. Behind the scenes, the drug companies have fought against "pot legalization;" BigPharma is unable to profit from cannabis, which cannot be patented because the plant is natural. Also, although the possession, growth and distribution of marijuana remains a felony under federal law, individual states and communities in the United States have bowed to the will of many people and some medical experts--who contend that cannabis has legitimate and necessary medical uses. Meantime, several states have legalized recreational marijuana, a trend that some observers expect to continue. The marijuana issue is only mentioned here as an example that although giant in size and rich, BigPharma is infallable, imperfect and the industry can sometimes "lose" on major issues. Thus, society should refrain from assuming that the drug industry will or should prevent certain types of medical robots that impact the sale and distribution of pharmaceuticals. For instance, consider the previously mentioned robots being designed to operate hospital pharmacies and to distribute drugs to patients within those facilities. If and when BigPharma is able to play a significant role in programming those machines, drug companies could very well accept and embrace such a transition. Pharmaceutical companies would be ensuring the continued sales of its products, while locking in profits.

Hospitals: Hospitals across the United States and the world already are grappling with the medical robotics issue. With cost-effectiveness a primary factor, administrators of medical facilities have been busy considering whether the expense of using robots will benefit these institutions. According to a June 2015 article in "Health Facilities Management Magazine," robots had recently joined medical personnel and general staff in greeting patients at the University of California San Francisco Medical School. The article said that 25 TUG-brand Robots at the facility spend a combined 350 hours every day tmaking about 1,300 trips and going a combined 481 miles in the facility. "The idea behind the robots is to free up employees from shuffling to and fro, when their time can instead be spent interacting with patients," the article said. "The robots handle such tasks

as transporting food, linens and specimens around the facility."
As previously mentioned, similar initial robotics systems were
already being gradually put into service at hospitals nationwide.
If the rollout and developments continued as projected, in steady
and progressive phases the vast majority of hospitals were to
have many of the high-tech robotics systems already described
in previous chapters. By early 2016 some hospitals already were
progressing much faster than other facilities in adopting robotics.
At UCSF Medical Center, for instance, the administration
had already started using a RIVA Machine(c), described as a
"robotic pharmacy" where the manmade devices coumpound
"chemotherapeutic drugs." If such devices are eventually deemed
as efficient and cost-effective enough to use a broad scale as
expected, other hospitals are likely to adopt similar technologies
by the mid-2020s. According to the article, at the San Francisco
hospital the robots had already produced up to 1.3 million doses
per year. Suzanne Leigh, a spokesman for the medical center, said
that the robotic pharmacy had made only one error, which resulted
from incorrect data that a person had input into the machinery.
"The robotic pharmacy reduces the potential for medication
errors," Leigh said. "It also frees up the pharmacist to spend more
time at the bedside discussing medication with the in-patient."
The article refrained from going into additional detail, primarily
the fact that the introduction of robotics into hospitals was steadily
accelerating nationwide. "Wired" Magazine has described such
devices as time- and cost-saving tools. Administrators at the San
Francisco medical center have been so impressed that they also
started using the robotic pharmacy to prepare oral and injectable
medicines. So, from the late 2010s and beyond, robots already
were "here to stay" in the American hospital industry.

     Politicians: Whether "political junkies" like to hear this
or not, the sad fact is that within the U.S. governmental system,
politicicians generally cater to the needs and wishes of those
who give them the biggest campaign donations. This likely
will hold true in regard to which new robotics systems will win

governmental approval. Under this line of thinking, whoever makes the largest donations has the greatest chance to "win." Although politicians are unlikely to consider each specific type of robotic system, these public servants could enact legislation regulating the overall "adoption process" of how robotics are introduced into the medical industry. In doing so, major or emerging robotics companies, hospitals and even BigPharma might get positioned for huge profits.

Health Care Professionals: Healthcare professionals ranging from nurses to technicians could soon see their livelihoods endangered; this will happen when hospitals and human doctors start using more specialized robots and other automated digital systems. The American Nurses Association acknowledged this trend in an article published on that organization's Website in May 2013. The story that emerging technologies will "change the practice of nursing." As a result, technology is transforming "the world at warp speed and nowhere is this more evident than healthcare settings." The story chronicles seven emerging technologies that will change nursing forever, plus new skills that these people will need in order to adapt to the expected transitions. Besides the introduction of robots into the medical industry, the other major listed new technologies are: computerized systems that make clinical decisions, in order to improve the efficiency of the ordering process and reduce "medical errors;" the startup and adoption of universal electronic medical records shared by all licensed healthcare providers; biometrics systems that increase the "security of confidental healthcare information;" a 3-D printing system, a revolutionary process that uses "bio-ink"--a mixture of living cells--used to create a "3-D structure of cells, layer-by-layer" to form human tissue and eventually human organs; less invasive medical tools for diagnostic and treatment, thereby reducing risk while lowering costs; and advances in genetics and genomics. As far as medical robotics, the Nursing Association acknowledged that the devices are designed to improve diagnostics while offering patients a more comfortable and less invasive experience. Yet it says that "more research is needed on the comparative effectiveness of robotics and healthcare providers. Many medical industry providers have expressed concern about the lack of emotion in robots, suggesting that this is the element that never will replace human caregivers." In reaching this conclusion, however, the well-intentioned people analyzing this transition apparently failed to take into account the fact that even by the late 2010s engineers had made tremendous progress in developing robots that seem--from the human perspective--to express and "show" emotion. Whether or not we humans like to acknowledge this, scientists had already started creating robots that display the characteristics of caring and empathy. These are the type of emotions that humans instinctively need and crave, particularly when ill or struggling to regain optimal health. So, perhaps the nurses' conclusions are somewhat self-serving, or at the very least "in denial about the truth regarding this all-encompassing transition."

Average people: The average person likely will have little or no say as to whether robots can or should be used in medical treatment and patient care.

First and foremost, typical "mere humans" lack the financial resources necessary to lauch and maintain any effective long-term and powerful political fight against the trend. Add to this the fact that most people lack any inkling that this transition is underway. As a result, upon entering hospitals or medical facilities as the years pass, most consumers will suddenly discover--often to their complete surprise--that this evolution has seemed to have "miraculously, mysteriously and suddenly occurred."

By that point, the vast majority of patients will find themselves in situations where they have no option other than to accept what already has transpired.

In many ways this will mirror the general public's reactions to new technologies that have been introduced during the past 120 years.

Left with little or no other options, for the most part

humans have embraced, accepted and quickly started using a vast range of "new-fangled" devices and medical techniques. These have ranged from TV sets and airplanes, to cars, telephones, cell phones, personal computers, hearing aids, heart pacemakers, and the Internet.

Prepare for the Unstoppable Outcome

Barring full-scale international war or a catastrophic event that destroys the economic infrastructure, in all likelihood medical robots will roll out into every sector of the medical industry.

Politicians, medical organizations, employee associations and hospitals ultimately will be able to do little or nothing to stop this transition.

In fact, quite disturbing from the viewpoint of many observers, robots will soon play a significant role in almost every aspect of our everyday lives. These new machine-based technologies will involve everything from transportation to our our households, and even how food is grown and distributed.

As you'll soon discover in subsequent chapters, universities, researchers, corporations and governments worldwide are actively working to make this all happen. Within the public mindset, on a worldwide scale, the "Rise of Robots" within medicine will become merely a "fascinating piece" of the big puzzle.

Whether or not we as a society collectively want to admit this, due to robotics the children born today will live as adults in a world far different from ours.

Prepare Mentally and Emotionally

Careful to keep these intertwined factors in clear focus, each of us needs to prepare for this unstoppable change on an emtoional and mental basis.

On the positive side, just based on what has been described to this point, you know far more about the issue at this critical juncture than the vast majority of people.

Right now, demographics experts say that more than 7 billion people are living worldwide, a number that continues to swell--without any sign of stalling.

This population expansion will test humanity's ultimate ability to effectively and efficiently use the earth's limited resources for the betterment of all mankind.

These developments, in turn, will force people to face two potential outcomes:

Robots will save humanity: Under this assumption, humans will depend on high-level robotics to save society from destruction. This theory concludes that humans are destroying the earth, causing so much pollution and chaos that only machines can safely and efficiently produce and distribute food, energy, people and products.

Robots will destroy humanity: Far stronger and much more intelligent than "mere humans," robots under this assumption will lead to the humanity's extinction. Some people fear that if robotic developments progresses as planned, the machines will be far "smarter" and much more powerful than "mere humans"--too dangerous to overcome.

Unpredictable Situation Prevails

The eventual impact of all types of robots remains impossible to predict, at least based on scientific reports, news articles and even declarations by some of the world's most famous people.

For instance, in mid-2015, world-famous scientists and entreprentuers declared that humanity faces extension due to robots and artificial intelligence.

Those issuing this urgent statement included: Stephen Hawking, an internationally acclaimed physist; Bill Gates, the founder of Microsoft; entrepeneur Elon Musk, a co-founder of PayPal and CEO of Tesla; and Steve Wozniak, instrumental in the startup of Apple computers.

Somewhat shockingly, most of the world seemed to treat

their mutual declaration as somewhat of an oddity.

American society seemed to greet their statement as if somewhat bizarre, almost as if these "brainiacks" were describing a far-out, theoretically impossible plot for a low-quality science fiction movie.

Everyone Should Pay Close Attention

Everyone needs to pay close attention to the issue, despite a rather blasé outlook by the general public. This holds true particularly through the initial rollout of robots through 2025.

The specific impact of robotics throughout the healthcare profession, and all other sectors of the economy, deserve intense public scrutiny.

Under ideal conditions, major public debates would be held on these related topics. Even so, such a fantasy dialogue likely will never occur on a massive scale.

For starters, the ill-informed public lacks any passion or intensity about robots.

So, you should never expect to hear adversaries argue these issues on the highest-rated live TV programs, situations that would generate huge ratings like the U.S. presidential debates.

Instead, pay close attention to the compelling robotics information that follows, to get an "insiders view" on the opinions of experts in business, economics and robotics.

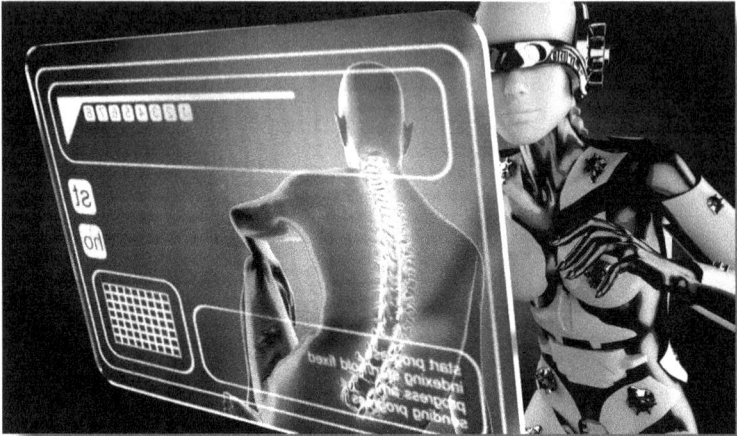

Chapter 12
Will Robots Replace Doctors?

An increasingly intense behind-the-scenes debate keeps erupting throughout the international medical community, which asks: "Will robots replace doctors?"

Rather than in public forums, most of these discussions or reports take place in scientific news stories and intermittent articles in medical publications.

While a limited number of doctors seem to discount the notion, many observers say "Yes," at least based on an unscientific survey of many of these articles.

"We need machines to make us smarter," Doctor Herbert Chase of the University of Columbia said in a "Ted Talk" presentation on the issue.

A professor of clinical medicine in biomedical informatics, Chase is among a growing number of medical experts who insist that this milestone transition will occur.

Physicians Use Known Data

Chase is among doctors who insist that no single human physician is smart enough to instantly calculate and make decisions based on all known medical data.

As proof, Chase emphasizes that doctors worldwide know of 13,000 diseases that people suffer; at least 6,000 medicines have been identified, created or approved.

Add to this the fact that physicians have developed 4,000 medical and surgical procedures, and the limitations of individual human doctors become evident.

Topping this off, thousands of data points or bits of information are involved in maintaining, inputting and anlyzing each person's medical record.

Yet on the positive side, according to the "Mobile

Health Global" publication, engineers have developed Artificial Intelligence that can instantly process the data.

Far More Efficient than Humans

The computer- and mechanical-based systems are able to instantly process and analyze data, automatically scanning thousands of complex medical reports.

Among people helping to lead the way is Doctor Bertalan Mesko, a medical futurist and author of "The Guide to the Future of Medicine."

Mesko insists that Artificial Intelligence, such as that used by advanced robots of the future, will initially enable human doctors to "make better decisions."

From Mesko's perspective, this factor in turn will enable healthcare professions to provide the absolute best therapy or treatment to patients after making a diagnosis.

Yet with equal emphasis some doctors have insisted that in order to achieve superior results, the process should involve far more than processing data.

Fine-Tune Robot Programming

"We need to learn to organize questions, so that we can exploit them and make them reliable," said Doctor Julio Mayol, as reported by the "Guide."

Mayol, a surgery professor and head of innovation at San Carlos Clinical Hospital in Madrid, Spain, insists that the infrastructure of the world's medical robotics system should be based on a specific model.

Just as essential, Mayol said, the data should enable the machines to make accurate findings, because "otherwise we'll get very precise (but) wrong conclusions."

Numerous medical publications and scientific articles emphasize the need for Artificial Intelligence or computer-based robotics to enable medical professionals to avoid making errors.

If such systems evolve as envisioned by electrical

engineers, the medical industry will eliminate the estimated 44,000 to 98,000 yearly deaths caused by negligence, at least from Mayol's view.

Critical Question Remains Unanswered

Although many doctors envision the need for enhanced computer-based data systems, the question of whether robots will replace doctors remains in dispute.

Chase is among doctors who insist that human physicians will remain irreplaceable, even if Artificial Intelligence advances as hoped by some medical experts.

Ideally, at least from the perspective of some observers the best outcomes will involve human doctors who use the projected technological advancements.

From the view of these experts, extremely "intelligent machines" could never possibly interact more effectively with patients than a human doctor.

To say otherwise likely would seem offensive or even outrageous, at least from the view of many of today's most respected, skilled and intelligent physicians.

The Blind Leading the Blind?

Any assumption that robots never could replace human doctors fails to take away the fact that engineers are developing robots identical to people.

The vast majority of us today have never seen only videos featuring the latest prototypes of "humanoids;" as previously mentioned, these robots look, behave and talk like humans.

The resemblance already is so uncanny--even in early prototypes--that telling the differences between some robots and actual humans seems difficult or even impossible.

"Keeping this factor in mind, who could possibly guarantee that machines never will replace human doctors?" some observers might ask. "Who can say for sure?"

Indeed, trying to accurately predict the entire medical

industry just 20 years from now would be like guaranteeing a 2051 Super Bowl outcome--"no one can say for sure."

Using Current Technology

With equal passion, some observers today might easily insist that current information-sharing systems can rapidly accelerate a doctor's decision-making process.

One of the most significant examples here involves the "Google Glass" product, eyeglasses that continually show the wearer images from the Internet.

When using these devices, a physician could easily and accurately scan the Web for necessary data--while also casually chatting with patients.

Such a procedure, in turn, would enable doctors to maintain and solidify the essential one-on-one relationship that they have with people who need their help.

Yet once again, this fails to take away the fact that engineers remain busy developing humanoids that are superior in intelligence and more durable than humans.

Business and Cost Factors

A wide variety of additional factors emerge, primarily involving why, how, when and where robots should replace doctors--plus what would make this happen:

Cost: The cost of building an individual robotic doctor, or RoboDoc, has not been announced. Yet presumably RoboDocs would be built on an assembly line, in much the way that cars are produced today. As a result, theoretically purchasing such a unit would be like going to a car dealership and purchasing your favorite model--for a flat fee.

Educational expenses: Each individual robot would not have to go through more than a decade of medical school and internship. Instead, the machines would be instantly programmed with all required information.

Re-education: Today's human doctors need continual

"re-education" or updates on the latest medical technology. This process is often time-consuming and expensive. By contrast, RoboDocs could instantly "learn" or be programmed with the latest info.

Hospital expenses: Rather than pay human doctors salaries or hourly fees that sometimes reach huge levels, hospitals and clinics would have a one-time purchase cost for each RoboDoc. The facilities likely would incur at least some maintenance expenses.

Retirement expenses: For their RoboDocs, hospitals and clinics never would have to contribute to retirement plans--the way that some facilities must do for human doctors. Instead, when "retirement" time comes for each RoboDoc, the hospital would simply ship the machine to a recycling facility that would crush the machine and recycle the materials.

Patient expenses: Exactly how much patient fees will get impacted remains a huge unknown factor. The medical facilities likely would want to keep these revenues, which otherwise would have gone to highly educated human medical professionals. (A subsequent chapter is devoted to the medical cost increases caused by robots and AI.)

Hospital motivation: Hospitals would use RoboDocs to cut employee expenses, thereby eliminating the supposed need for human doctors, while also striving to improve efficiency and eliminate errors.

Triggers for Change
All these various transitions that bring RoboDocs into the medical system will hinge on political, business, technological and economic factors.

For hospital administrators to eventually erect the proverbial green "go" flag allowing all this to happen, they first must be convinced of the cost benefit.

Obviously, none of these changes will occur until the ideal, effective and easy-to-manage technology becomes available;

93

approval only will come if authorities conclude that RoboDocs or less advanced medical robots provide superior medical care.

Then, there also are the previously mentioned political factors that eventually must all line up in favor of bringing these machines into the fold.

Remember the aforementioned fact that the Almighty Dollar will remain the primary motivating factor, rather than merely trying to improve patient health.

Additional Factors Emerge

The various factors already described that impact doctors also will effect additional healthcare professionals--from pharmacists to nurses.

Once again, medical facility administrators will consider various criteria when deciding whether to replace these healthcare industry professionals with machines.

The matter of labor unions would emerge, particularly involving nurses. All of these professionals might lose their jobs to robots or advanced software, eliminating the viability of these employees' unions.

Such outcomes, in turn, would sharply decrease or even fully eliminate the personnel expenses that medical facilities now must pay on an ongoing basis.

Would such changes free up funds for additional medical research? Or, in a more likely scenario, would various corporations benefit from increased stock prices, while doing little to improve health care?

Consider the "Human Toll"

All of these issues collectively generate a formidable paradox.

By adopting robots in efforts to improve health care, medical facilities would decimate or destroy numerous viable, worthy and distinguished professions.

Just as confusing, while striving to help patients with

significant technological advancements, these businesses would destroy many livelihoods.

In a broad sense, hospitals and clinics would inflict economic suffering on their former employees--all apparently, or at least hopefully--while patients benefit by living longer and healthier lives. Such conclusions assume that medical robots will be far more efficient than human healthcare professionals.

These various considerations would, in turn, cause a potentially disastrous ripple effect. Think of the potential harm or changes to medical schools, nursing schools and a maze of businesses that serve those institutions.

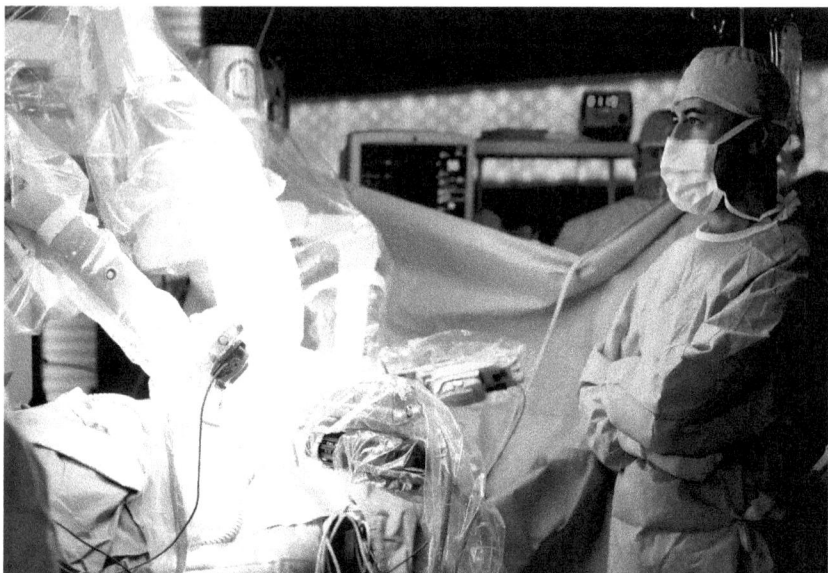

Chapter 13
The Transition Has Begun Toward Medical Robots

Like this or not, the transition of robots into hospitals has alrady begun.

"Robots are increasingly finding themselves employed in clinical environments, where their orderliness and detachment are prized skills," Chandra Steel said in an April 2015 article in "PC Magazine."

"They've started with handing out pills and dispensing meals," Steel said. "And, one robot even performs surgery with the assistance of a real, carbon-based surgeon. But it's possible that a robot might one day be making medical assessments on its own."

Steel's article lists seven robots that already assist human doctors:

Watson: This IBM "wonderbot" is helping doctors treat cancer patients, enabling oncologists to use DNA-based treatments for the most common type of brain cancer, glioblastoma. Determined to effectively treat this ailment that kills 13,000 Americans yearly, human doctors use Watson to correlate massive amounts of data.

Da Vinci Surgical System: Using tiny precision tools, these robots assist human surgeons with minimally invasive surgeries. The machines use a "controller" to carry out the human physician's movements, while the system provides the doctor with a 3D and HD view of the surgery. Thanks to this efficient system, according to engineers, the patients enjoy a faster recovery time while suffering less trauma. Yet "PC Magazine" lists this system as possibly "imperfect," noting that the device had been named in numerous lawsuits.

Remote assessments: InTouch TeleStroke Solution robots enable doctors to remotely visit and assess the conditions of stroke patients. By "remotely," this means the physician who specializes in strokes might be in New York City, while the patient is in a hospital bed in a remote rural community such as Ely, Nevada. After assessing the patients via video hookups and video screens, in this example, these specialists then communicate with and give advice to human doctors at the Ely hospital. Medical experts deem this system as particularly helpful to patients and doctors in rural areas. (These are somewhat similar to the previously mentioned "telerobots."

Receptionists: Robots already are working as receptionists and greeters at numerous hospitals in Japan, where the senior population is growing much faster than that nation's sluggish birth rate. Lacking enough young people to fill the receptionist jobs, hospital administrators in Japan have eagerly started using the robots. If these initial prototypes prove successful, other hospitals worldwide likely will start using similar machines as a cost-saving measure; this would eliminate personnel expenses.

Heavy lifting: Steadily increasing numbers of U.S. hospitals, and medical facilities elsewhere, already were using TUG-brand robots to transport heavy or light-weight objects and materials to various locations throughout those buildings. Items range from meals to linens, medication and laboratory specimens.

SimMan G3: These name-brand robots simulate human patients. Medical students and new doctors undergoing "residency" use these specialized machines to simulate actual medical conditions amid training. This helps the learning process considerably because the devices accurately mimic actual patients. Besides vocalizing their "distress," these robots realistically react to medications and display information detailing physiological symptoms.

Dispensing drugs: The Robot RX-brand machine, developed by Aesynt, can fill most prescriptions within hospitals, even "deciding" the appropriate treatments and dosages for patients. According to the "PC Magazine" article, the machine can: create medications on site; free up human pharmacists for other tasks; streamline dispensation; and even "work on clinical drug trials."

Human joints: Some doctors already are using the trademarked and specialized Rio Robotic Arm Interactive Orthopaedic System. The devices improve the function of damaged hip or knee joints by resurfacing those natural structures. Doctors work with the Rio robots in performing "Makoplasty" procedures, striving to minimize or eliminate the negative symptoms of osteoarthritis.

Debate Erupts Among Physicians

At a steadily increasing pace in recent years some human doctors have cringed at scientific predictions that robots could eventually replace them.

In a September 2012 article for "Imaging Technology News," medical industry consultant Greg Freiherr gave a clear and concise analysis of the situation.

Freiherr noted that a founder of Sun Microsystems, Vinod Khosla, had predicted that computer-based decisions based on patient data would "lead to better health care" than provided by human doctors.

Khosla said that under this scenario robotics systems would provide objective analysis, unlike human physicians whom he claims arguably have hackneyed ways of thinking and embedded procedures.

As a result, Freiherr's article said, this "led Khosla to conclude that at least 80 percent of doctors could be replaced by software."

Machines Verses Humans

Physicians and medical professionals wage a daily battle against this kind of thinking, according to Freiherr. As an example, he noted that radiologists strive to reduce their patients' exposure to a known cardinogen, radiation.

Some Emergency Room doctors order computer-based tomography (CT) scans of children who suffer minor injuries. This happens even though merely observing the patient for several hours has proven just as effective, Freiherr said.

He suggests that in such instances doctors sometimes order potentially dangerous tests out of fear of potential litigation, rather than using a common-sense approach.

"When combined with love for a child who we fear may be severely hurt, it's damn the radiation--fire up the CT," Freiherr said.

"In Khosla's future, machines would call the shots; their decisions would be based on algorhythms. Some would argue current-day health care already is. Diagnosticians are taught to think horses, not zebras; to consider common ailments before rare ones."

Differences in "Logic"

As noted by Freiherr, humans can strive for a common-sense approach, such as radiologists ordering less dangerous ultrasound or MRI procedures whenever possible.

Under Khosla's vision, machines would process information using a level of objectivity unattainable by humans. Robots ideally would base their objectivity on data, a "machine-based logic" that sharpens with experience.

Unlike people, the robots never would have to overcome love when making life-and-death decisions; the machines would avoid making fear-based choices.

From this perspective, such cold-hearted objectivity could eventually enable robots to improve the overall practice of medicine.

Freiherr is among healthcare experts who agree that such logic might improve health care--but only when such interpretations are "applied by caring doctors."

Ultimately, he argues, medicine involves truly caring for people, not just individuals whose illnesses can be determined and cured. This contrasts with the cold-hearted approach, which ignores the urgent and passionate human emotions that motivate patients to fight onward; such heart-felt emotion often generates a passionate survival mode that gives patients the determination that is necessary to persevere through seemingly insurmountable situations.

Critics Voice Concerns
In an October 2015 article in the "Telegraph," Jessica Powell asks readers to envision a GP surgery in the future.

Under this scenario, Powell says, a robot with a super-computer brain calculates drug doses in mere seconds--never bogged down by possible fatigue-induced errors.

Based on ongoing advancements in Artificial Intelligence, Powell declares that such a scene might seem possible--especially amid shortages in qualified personnel.

Yet Powell quoted the chairman at the University of Warwick, Richard Lilford, as convinced that actual situations such as these never will occur.

Powell summarizes Lilford's statements by proclaiming that anyone who thinks otherwise would be grossly underestimating the complex skills of human doctors.

Going for the Proverbial Juggler
"I'm a sceptic on Artificial Intelligence," Powell quoted Lilford as saying. "I don't think computers will ever supplant the doctor's diagnosis. I think things will change--I think computers might suggest a diagnosis."

Lilford cites situations where a computer or robot might fail to notice--or to factor in--critical and necessary information when making a diagnosis.

As an example Lilford describes a situation where a doctor treats a patient who has just returned from a visit to India, where dangerous dengue fever commonly spreads.

A computer might motivate the doctor to consider such

facts when reaching a diagnosis. But Lilford predicts that "the doctor will still make the final call."

Among the numerous critical factors Lilford mentions:

Certainty: Robots are programmed to process known facts, basing their calculations or decision-making process on "certainty." Yet human doctors have and need the ability to make quick judgments, often before all potentially revelant details are determined. The machines lack the unique human ability to rely on intuition.

Bedside manner: Human doctors also have the unique ability to show genuine empathy for patients, another essential factor that Lilford believes robots lack. He views the separation of psychological and human care as "lethal"--largely because robots invariably fail to display or feel genuine compassion.

Counter Arguments

Powell's article never mentions the fact that by late 2015, according to numerous news reports, scientists had successfully uploaded human personalities into robots.

Perhaps just as compelling came news that biologists and engineers had also developed technology to upload data from living human brains into machines.

While failing to recognize or acknowledge such landmark developments, are many of today's medical experts essentially burying their heads in the sand on this issue?

Are adversaries of medical robotics merely behaving like ostriches, or should observations such as Lilford's play a greater role in the development of these machines?

From my view, the overall success or failure of the integration of robotics into medicine will come down to these urgent and unavoidable factors:

Patients: Would patients emotionally and physically accept such treatment?

Robots: Will engineers develop robots that behave and appear human, capable of displaying a sense of genuine emotion necessary to optimize treatment--while gaining the essential trust of patients?

Results: Can and will robots help patients as well as--or better than--human doctors?

Costs: Briefly mentioned earlier, will RoboDoctors increase hospital profits, while also minimizing patient expenses?

At this critical juncture in the ongoing development of such devices, robotic engineers seem optimistic. Yet taking a sharply different position, many of us within the medical profession remain understandably pessimistic.

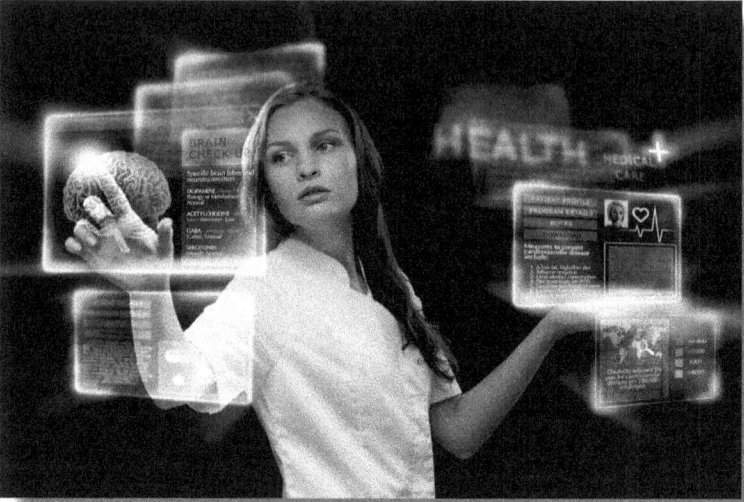

Chapter 14
Will People Accept Medical Robots?

Of significant importance on an international scale, the milestone development of medical robots hinges on the effectiveness of these devices and whether people accept the machines.

These factors bring forth critical questions. How, why and where people will allow themselves to get medical treatment from "mere robots" remains unknown.

If recent history serves as an indicator, in all probability humans will either eagerly or at least willingly accept--and even feel dependent on--such technology.

Assuming this happens, could the healthcare industry reach a point where only a handful of people would proclaim, "I refuse to ever get medical checkups from robots, or to be treated by such machines?"

Despite such logical declarations, if advancements continue as engineers plan, people will have no option other than to accept robotic medical treatment when seeking professional health care.

Most People "Do What You Tell Them to Do"

For the most part, the bulk of society has readily accepted streams of new medical techiques and systems during the past century.

"Wow! How did they do that!" many people seemed to think when these transitions occurred. "What in the world will they think of next? This is amazing."

From the discovery of a vaccine as a cure for polio and beyond, for the most part people have unquestioningly embraced anything that extends or improves life.

These rapidly advancing systems have often resulted in

reductions in medical fees, improved health, increased efficiency and saved time for patients and medical experts.

One of the most significant accomplishments came in the 1950s when streams of families flocked to public buildings to get polio vaccinations. Back then, most U.S. citizens complied with a government mandate that everyone get such innoculations.

Social Media Breeds Protests

Despite the willingness over many generations of people to accept new medical technology, advances in information-sharing platforms, social media services and texting have made such efforts more difficult for the public to accept.

Indeed, the overall issue of medical robots is likely to take on a more controversial aura due to social media, which was non-existent in the mid-20th Century.

Using these technologies that were unavailable more than 50 years ago, the bulk of today's population is able to band together in criticizing government policies or new healthcare devices.

A key example involves the controversial use and mandatory innoculations of children to prevent many diseases. Some parents have protested throughout the most popular social media platforms; these critics insist that such medications have sharply increased the nationwide rate of autism.

The resulting dispute has intensified the political and social battles between some parents and the medical industry. Most doctors and scientists insist that innoculations are harmless, while a fraction of parents say otherwise; many of these criticisms come from people who lack any medical expertise.

This dispute, in turn, has led to instances where some people discussing this issue via social media resort to childish name-calling. Such arguments occasionally erupt when people describe anyone who disagrees with them as "crazies," "whackos," or even "insane."

People Want Scientific Proof

Largely due to today's instant, high-tech communication systems, a sector of today's society seems less prone to accept everything that the government proclaims.

This marks a significant change from the 1940s and 1950s, when only a handful of people generated widespread publicity when protesting government policies regarding health care.

In a sharp turn-around from that era, today's consumers have greater power in demanding scientific proof when officials impose societal changes.

Partly for these reasons, the term "question authority" has become increasingly popular. Even so, precisely how such protests might impact the Rise of Medical Robots remains a big unknown.

Perhaps hospitals and medical clinics will start using the machines much sooner than many people realize, before the general public has a chance to launch protests powerful enough to stop or delay such transitions.

Hoping for such an outcome, perhaps robotics industry officials and people allied to them will adopt these technologies seemingly in "the blink of an eye;" healthcare facilities would strive to start using the new systems long before most consumers realize what has been happening.

Wide-Scale Acceptance Already Exists

Consumers worldwide, and particularly in the United States, have eagerly accepted significant new medical technologies on a massive scale in recent decades.

A non-scientific review of media reports indicate there have been little or no protests. The public remained relatively quiet, even in the wake of significant discoveries or inventions that forever changed the medical industry.

From among many dozens of improvements made possible by biomedical engineering, some of the most publicized advancements have been:

Organ transplants: Unheard of and seemingly unimaginable several decades ago, these procedures have become relatively commonplace in industrialized countries. Heart, lung or kidney transplants have extended life for thousands of people.

Natural remedies: Although somewhat controversial among mainstream doctors, my West Coast clinic uses an effective protocol of natural remedies and standard medicine. Remember the aforementioned fact that advanced Stage IV cancer patients treated at my clinic have nearly a 33 times greater chance of survival, as compared to similar patients who are treated by "mainstream oncologists." (You can review these essential details in a Bonus Section near the end of this book.)

Open-heart surgeries: Rarely performed and often unsuccessful just a century ago, these operations have become fairly routine in recent decades. Scientists say a fairly good success rate has resulted in widespread public acceptance of these procedures.

Laser surgeries: Virtually unheard of for the most part as recently as the 1980s, operations that involve lasers also have become relatively common--even in non-hospital, clinical settings. These procedures on everything from eyes to gums and internal organs have greatly improved results, while accelerating recovery time.

Along with many other new medical advancements, too numerous to mention in full, new technologies such as these have almost invariably been accepted by consumers.

Robots Present Unique Challenges

By delving into an all-new universe of medical advancements, robots are likely to pose unique challenges on the human psyche--unlike the other improvements.

To help put this into perspective, consider the following scenario--which could click into gear within 20 years if the technology progresses as planned.

Under such a revamped medical industry infrastructure,

you are checked into a hospital where most or all "medical professionals" are actually robots.

Would you protest, saying that "I refuse to be diagnosed and treated by machines?" Or, would you accept all this, saying "let us do what needs to be done?"

Well, like this or not, under such a scene you invariably would have no option other than to allow robots to treat you-- unless humans successfully require that "licensed human medical professionals be involved."

Would Robots "Put You Under the Knife?"

Many of the most perplexing issues facing individual human patients likely will involve a "fear of the unknown," particularly amid initial stages of this transition.

How would you react when surrounded by robotic medical professionals--without any people present other than you?

Imagine the machines telling you, "We need to operate on your internal organs. Please sign this document allowing us to proceed with the surgery."

If you refuse to authorize the operation, at least under this scenario, in all likelihood there would be no experienced or licensed human doctors capable of peforming the procedure for you.

Worsening matters, if you reject the robotic surgery, these machines might have to follow a protocol requiring your discharge from the hospital or medical facility. Under such worst-case situations this might require you to "go home and wait to die."

Trickle-Down Process

Well before such worries can erupt on a massive scale, robotics companies and doctors are either unintentionally or purposefully engaging in a unique and mind-boggling transition strangely called a "trickle-down upgrade."

This involves gradually introducing robots into hospitals and medical clinics worldwide. In some instances this already is occurring on an increasingly massive scale, as the vast majority of consumers fail to realize that these changes are happening.

Largely as a result, there seems to have been little or absolutely no public protests or wide-scale complaints.

At least judging from news reports on these "upgrades," patients or even medical professionals have readily accepted these critical changes.

During these early stages, initial versions of medical robotics have ranged from the previously mentioned doctor-assisted machines that do "rounds" at patient rooms, to surgical devices used remotely by physicians and the "robot pharmacies."

Adjusting the Public Mindset

Chances seem strong that advanced medical industry machines including robots have been readily accepted by patients primarily because these people find themselves "left with no other option."

Many consumers live in communities where the only available hospitals or health clinics already have the devices.

This trend should intensify as steadily increasing numbers of "non-intelligent, non-medical robots" are used in such facilities. Commonly called "domestic robots," these previously mentioned machines handle cleaning, maintenance and other basic duties such as receptionist tasks.

Largely as a result, at least to this point, the use of robotic devices in health care facilities has failed to emerge into a widely debated hot-button issue.

Meantime, particularly through around 2025, the early stages of medical robotics likely will involve only "non-thinking" machines without computer-based brains. Designed primarily to perform automated tasks that never involve decisions, the domestic robots likely will increase the public's acceptance of such devices in medical environments.

This transition should "set the stage," mentally preparing the public for the critical period from 2025 to 2035 when the medical industry's extensive robotics upgrades are expected to click into full gear--at least if engineers reach their goals by then.

Subsequently, if researchers keep these advancements on track, starting more than a decade from now consumers will find themselves with no option other than to allow autonomous robots to make healthcare decisions.

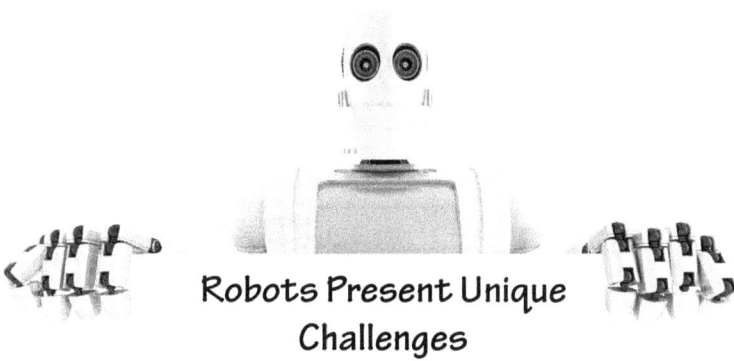

Robots Present Unique Challenges

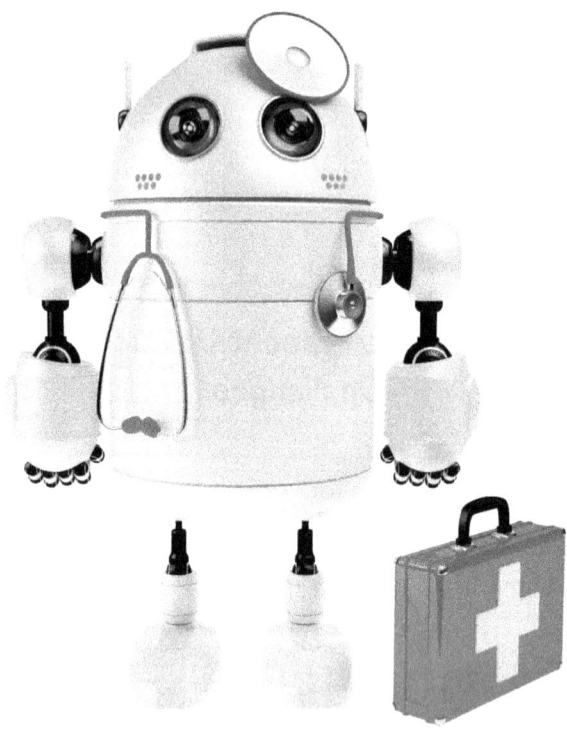

Robots to the Rescue?

Chapter 15
Human Doctors Face Extreme Challenges

The movement of robotics into the medical industry comes at a pivotal time, when increasing numbers of doctors want to leave their profession.

This comes as little surprise because individual physicians are expected to achieve and maintain a super-human level of performance.

"With a growing, aging population, the demand for physicians has intensified, and communities around the country already are experiencing doctor shortages," says a statement posted on the Website of the Association of American Medical Colleges (AAMC).

By 2025, the United States will have 46,000 to 90,000 fewer doctors than needed, according to a study conducted by IHS Inc.

"The shortages pose a real risk to patients," the assocation said. "Because it takes between five to 10 years to train a doctor, projected shortages in 2025 will need to be addressed so that patients will have acccess to the care they need."

Robots to the Rescue?

Medical associations refrained from recommending that RoboDoctors fill the gap.

Instead, some organizations propose that medical professionals develop systems that enable human physicians to work better together in teams.

This strategy would join physicians with a variety of other healthcare experts in a joint effort to increase efficiency. Yet even the medical college organization agrees that such systems would fail to correct the growing and critically important problem of doctor shortages.

The assocation suggests that Congress proceed with proposals to allow medical schools to train 3,000 more new doctors yearly. To do this, lawmakers would have to lift a cap on federally funded residency training positions.

Amid these challenges, numerous physicians' organizations have become increasingly worried that proposed cutbacks in college funding would worsen the problems.

Obamacare and Bureaucracy Exacerbate These Challenges

Many people failed to notice, but as medical robotics research intensified, increasing numbers of doctors decided to quit the profession--because of Obamacare, which formally has a propaganda-based name, the "Affordable Health Care Act."

Numerous liberal analysts insisted that these problems were never happening. But the indisputable, cold-hard facts indicated otherwise. Among the many reasons:

Bureaucracy: Some doctors announced their decision to quit the profession because Obamacare resulted in mounds of unnecessary--but required--paperwork.

Quality: Frustrated physicians said Obamacare created a sharp reduction in the overall quality of patient care, an overly bureaucratic system that ignores patient needs.

Politicians: Politicians and bureaucrats with no medical training were making critical decisions on patient care; this prevents doctors from providing the best services.

Catastrophic Industry Flip-Flops Accelerated

The decision by Congress to essentially tie up the entire medical industry with bureaucratic red tape came as research into medical robotics intensified.

According to a "Daily Caller" report in June 2012, by that time a whopping 83 percent of all U.S. doctors had considered quitting due to Obamacare.

Nearly two years after this controversial survey, many doctors had made a final decision to leave their profession, according the "Reporting on Health" publication.

That story published in March 2014 noted that of all practicing doctors then, one out of every four doctors would reach retirement age by 2019.

The posting by R. Jan Gurley quoted a 22-year pediatrician as saying that in Contra Costa Country, California, "many doctors have left and all are considering leaving" due to the issues imposed by government regulations.

Is this "The Perfect Storm?"

These challenging issues might have created a "perfect storm," the mass exodus of human doctors from their profession-- amid the increasingly intense development and rollout of medical robots.

As if to underscore this trend, without mentioning robots, in a 2013 Deloitte survey of 20,000 physicians, 62 percent of the doctors predicted that they would retire earlier than planned-- perhaps within the next one to three years.

"This perception is fairly uniform among all physicians, irrelevant of age, gender and medical specialty," the Deloitte report said.

Perhaps even more disturbingly, nearly six out of every 10 doctors answered a survey question by saying the "practice of medicine is in jeopardy."

Some analysts insisted that bureaucratic requirements increased the workload of doctors whose practices involve medical specialties. Government-mandated paperwork intensified as some specialists got stuck with reimbursement rates much lower than in other sectors of the medical industry.

Filling the "Gap" Imposes Challenge

Filling the proverbial "hole in the dike," the projected shortage in human doctors becomes even more of a challenge amid the current high-tech "information age."

While deciding which professions to eventually enter,

teenagers in high school or young adults in college might want to avoid medicine.

Will increasing numbers of prospective doctors shun the medical industry, concentrating on potentially lucrative professions that involve robotics?

Upon discovering that prospective or current doctors are "getting a raw deal," qualified students might flock to the burgeoning robotics industry.

Rather than apply for medical school or take undergraduate courses leading to such schooling, students would "go where the big money and growth has started to flow--and that is robots."

These courses range from physics and mathematics to metallugry, each leading to potential jobs in robotics or business sectors related to that industry.

Why Enter a Dying Profession?

If many business analysts, robotics experts and futurists are correct, anyone entering medical school today gets positioned for an overall "dying" profession.

By comparison, for the past several hundred years, society and investors have considered the ownership and operation of newspapers as an "enterprise industry." Such businesses were considered as "evergreen," meaning that they would remain rock-solid and profitable for thousands of years--a so-called permanent bedrock for society.

The Internet, social media and instant communications changed all that. Since the mid-1990s newspaper stocks have slumped amid a nose-dive in readership. To counteract this trend, which came as a shock to many longtime newspaper executives, those businesses now strive to remain relavent by integrating with social media.

Transitions such as these generate a maze of complex and intriguing questions for anyone already in--or amid the process of entering--the medical or robotics professions.

Once again all of society faces a nagging but necessary

dilemma, namely the pivotal challenge of how the healthcare industry, medical schools and doctors will adapt to the Rise of the Robots.

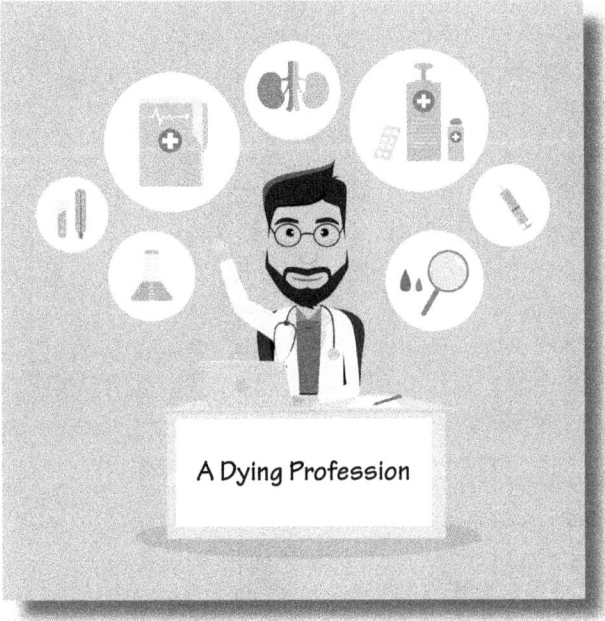

A Dying Profession

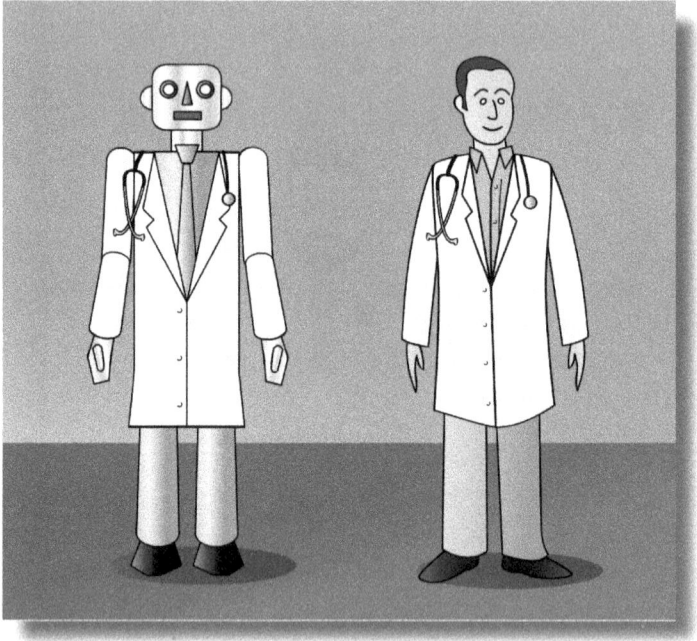

Chapter 16
Compare Robots to Human Doctors

The many complex and intermingled issues of medical robotics ultimately lead to the obvious need to compare the general attributes and differences between robots and human doctors.

How would these characteristics compare with each other, everyhing from stamina and knowledge, to the capability to handle an intense work load?

What follows is a hypothetical, non-scientific comparsion. These examples are based on my many years of extensive experience as a practicing doctor, plus various news and scientific reports about advancements in medical robotics. These examples also assume the RoboDocs and human doctors work full-time.

In addition, under this scenario the human doctor is a family practitioner, a specialist in internal medicine or a primary care physician. This person works daily, with no days off, while maintaining weekday office hours. Meantime, the RoboDoc used in this hypothetical scenario operates 24 hours daily, every day. Here are the comparisons:

Stamina

Human doctor: The human doctor works an exhausting schedule, from eight to 10 hours daily in the office, plus an additional 1-2 hours daily in hospitals or nursing homes. This person is continually overworked, striving to manage personal stress and with little time to pursue a fulfilling personal life.

Robot: The machine "works" 24 hours daily, 365 days a year without needing breaks--except for occasional brief time off for mechanical maintenance.

Personal Interruptions

Human doctor: Throughout an entire medical career, this

person struggles for personal time off. This individual strives to engage in "normal" family activities such as birthdays, holiday meals, attending children's school events, and having a fulfilling relationship with a spouse, lover or other relatives.

Robot: Has absolutely no need or desire for "personal life," so family issues are non-existent. As a result, the machine can dedicate every moment to medical care, without having to engage in family-oriented activities.

Early-morning Responsibilities

Human doctor: Each work day starts out hectic, even before patients arrive. From 8-9 a.m., the physician keeps busy: reviewing lab reports and X-rays; communicating with hospitals and nursing homes for updates on individual patients and related issues; returning phone calls; and completing necessary medical reports.

Robot: The robot never has to "do these tasks" on such a pre-set schedule; instead, such chores are automatically done non-stop on a 24-hour basis. This happens automatically thanks to constant Internet communications, which sends data via Wi-Fi into the machine's "computer-based brain"--while also sharing information with others.

Brief Work Break

Human doctor: Striving to remain energized and mentally sharp, from 9:00 to 9:15 a.m., the physician takes a coffee or juice break.

Robot: No break is necessary; this gives the machine more time than the human for "working" on patient care.

The Day's First Patient

Human doctor: From 9:15-9:30, the physician has a follow-up patient meeting. After reviewing the person's medical chart, the doctor spends 6 or 7 minutes visiting the person. The physician then issues prescriptions, orders necessary lab or

X-ray work, and completes an Electronic Medical Records report required by the government.

Robot: Unlike the 15 minutes required by the human doctor, the machine needs only 5 minutes to interact with the patient, order necessary tests or drugs, and complete paperwork. Such efficiency enables the machine to visit with three follow-up patients in every 15-minute period, compared to just one person during similar time frames for the human doctor.

First-Time Patient

Human doctor: From 9:30-10:15 a.m., the doctor sees a new patient. The 45-minute examination is three times longer than the standard 15-minute check-up that returning patients receive. During this initial visit the physician spends 15 or 20 minutes reviewing the person's medical history; another 20 minutes is dedicated to a thorough examination. This involves everything from the breast and pelvic area, to a rectal exam and the prostate or other organs. Then, the doctor performs two more separate exams of new patients; these are 45-minute sessions from 10:15 to 11, and 11 to 11:45.

Robot: Unlike the 45-minute exams of new patients that the human doctor performs, the robot only needs from 5 minutes to 10 minutes to perform each of these procedures. This is possible because the robot has: instant information "memorized" or stored on the patient's entire medical history; high-tech, non-invasive scanning devices perform the first-time patient, in-office exams in less than a few minutes. At the end of each session, the RoboDoc gives the patient a thorough printout of examination results.

Time Comparison

Through the morning, the human doctor performed thorough examinations of three new or first-time patients during a 2-hour, 15-minute period. By comparison, the robot visited at least 13 new patients, and possibly even more. Upon leaving their first-time examinations, the people who visited the human doctor had been given basics regarding their prognosis; most of these patients learn that they will have to wait several days for more conclusive test results. Yet patients visiting the robot for the first time get a much different experience. Firstly, the machine provides the thorough initial diagnosis briefly mentioned earlier. And, secondly, immediately after the robot leaves this session, "counselors" that are either human or machines interact and communicate with the patient. This is done to teach or counsel the patient, answer all questions that the individual has; and to give instructions on what the patient should do during treatments--details such as taking medications, or preparing for any necessary surgery.

Hectic Lunchtime Routine

Human doctor: Many people in the western culture, particularly within the United States, prefer to enjoy their lunch breaks during the noon hour. Yet under this scenario based on real-life situations, a human physician in family practice, internal medicine or primary care must juggle a maze of essential responsibilities. Under this scenario the doctor works non-stop from 11:45 a.m to 12:50 p.m. signing and reading paperwork, and returing patients' phone calls.

Robot: The robot never has to spend time reading and signing paperwork. Those tasks are handled either automatically by this primary machine, or by other robotic devices used as "assistants." The patients phone calls are handled automatically by "electronic voices" that talk to the people; the information that these automated machines provide verbally is instantly inputted into the computer-based system--every word.

Hectic or Efficient Afternoons

Human doctor: Lacking time for a decent lunch, the physician seizes any available moment for food brought from home or purchased in the hospital or clinic. Some doctors manage to schedule 45-minute lunch breaks. Most afternoons are typically spent doing non-stop, 15-minute patient follow-up visits. This

entails at least 10 such sessions through 4 o'clock in the afternoon-
-often with at least one first-time patient examination during that
period.

Robot: During this period when the human doctor would
have seen about 10 follow-up patients, the robot is able to serve
from 30 to 50 people. This sharply increases the hospital or
clinic's perceived efficiency--at much less expense than paying a
human doctor.

Necessary Late-afternoon Tasks

Human doctors: The late afternoons and early evenings
are spent on vital, essential and sometimes cumbersome tasks.
From 4-4:45, the doctor needs to complete charts, government-
mandated reports, and review lab and X-ray results. The non-stop
work continues from 4:45-5:45 as the physician visits patients
in hospitals and nursing homes, or spends much of that time
returning phone calls. Then, from 5:45-6:45 the doctor has vital
meetings or discussions with staffers or other physicians in these
various healthcare facilities.

Robots: Similar to what already has occurred during
the noon hour, the robot or other "assistant" machines already
have automatically performed all paperwork. On a continual,
24-hour basis all patient test results are automatically uploaded
into the robot's computer-based "brain" or memory system. So,
this machine does not need to spend time reviewing laboratory or
X-ray results. The robot never attends meetings with staffers or
other health care professionals at hospitals or nursing homes; those
communications are handled automatically via instantaneous and
continual Web-based communications--even while the machines
or human health care professionals are physically located in
different buildings. In addition, the robot never needs to travel to
the various healthcare facilities to visit patients. The in-hospital or
nursing home visits are done by similar robots--which each have
received the same automatically uploaded data on each patient.

Challenging Rest and Relaxation Time

Human doctor: Mirroring an arduous process that began during medical school, the doctor struggles to get adequate rest and family time. At the height of the doctor's career, the phone often rings in the middle of the night; answering services convey details about round-the-clock patient inquiries. The physician fails to get adequate sleep, returing patient phone calls at all hours. Meantime, some of the doctor's family relationships get tested as a result, amid occasional allegations from spouses or relatives that "you were never there for me when I needed you. Why are your patients more important to you than I am? Why can't you just slow down your career, and spend quality time with people who love you?" Yet no matter how well-intentioned the doctor might be, any effort to increase family time--while also striving to maintain a professional medical practice--becomes a formidable challenge.

Robot doctor: Although programmed to display emotions such as empathy or even humor, the machine has no "personal" family responsibilities. Any necessary call-backs to patients during the late-night or wee-morning hours are made by automated systems that share data from an informational medical database.

"Free Time" During Off Hours

Human doctor: As previously mentioned, the person struggles to get adequate rest while remaining well-nourished, particularly during rare or infrequent time "away from work."

Robot: Without a "worry in the world," the machine is "off duty" whenever the clinic or medical practice is closed. Early-version robots will be plugged in for battery recharging, before subsequent updated models continually recharge themselves with light; this eliminates any need to stop "work" in order to schedule or accommodate for re-charging time.

Staffing Requirements

Human doctor: Under this scenario, the physician maintains a four-person staff plus at least one nurse and an office manager. All medical practices have extensive costs that include: rent or mortgage; medical equipment; licensing, uniforms, pharmaceuticals; and business insurance. Managing and tracking these various expenses and necessary infrastructure becomes a monumental task, especially for large individual medical practices. Per-patient charges vary from $1,000 to $1,400 for first-time visits, to $250 to $400 for follow-ups. Per-day staff pay sometimes reaches $640 daily for the combined four staffers at $20 hourly, and also $640 daily for the combined salaries of the nurse and manager at $40 per hour. Topping this off, at least under this example, janitorial fees reach about $1,580 per week. Various medical industry reports and news stories list vastly different estimates on the average annual income of U.S. doctors. Many published estimates seem to range from about $150,000 to $300,000. While this might seem high from the perspective of most people, many physicians keep themselves and their families in far too much debt. As a result, human physicians who fail to save sometimes "barely make ends meet" from month-to-month, while never accumulating the necessary funds for retirement. These factors, in turn, sometimes increase the stress levels of individual human doctors.

Robot: In all likelihood, the machine will not own or even personally oversee the management of the clinic, medical practice or hospital where the device "works." At least under this scenario, the profitability of the facility will never be among the primary functions for which the robot has been programmed. At this early juncture, before such advanced units go into "service," any projection of facility revenues and patient costs would only be mere "pie-in-the-sky" forecasts. The machines only handle patient care, rather than needing to concentrate on profitability or revenue-generation.

Respect from the Public
Human doctors: The vast majority of today's human doctors get little or no respect from the general public, particualy

when compared to the mid-20th Century. Rather than refer to their physicians as "doctor," increasing percentages of today's patients casually refer to their physicians by first name. I remember the 1960s and 1970s, when the vast majority of patients respectfully listened to their physicians; patients latched on to every word from medical professionals. For the most part patients back then adhered to every recommendation made by their doctors. Today, in a sharp reversal, increasingly large percentages of patients are argumentative--"difficult to deal with." Perhaps this flagrant disrespect comes from our changing cultural practices, where some consumers whine and complain about virtually everything they encounter. The advent of social media has worsened this situation. On public "ratings" Websites, consumers gripe about everything from what "they think that they have been told," to their assessment of how a specific procedure was performed. Topping this off, some consumers post blatant assessments online, overly critical about the bedside manner of individual doctors. As a result, human physicians who work non-stop trying to build positive reputations for themselves and for their medical practices often find themselves "beaten down" in the public arena.

Robots: Machines specializing in medicine or healthcare treatment likely will become the target of intense public criticisms as well. When this happens, the people who build or program these robots can choose to update the existing devices with new specifications and operations critria--or build all-new models. Consumers and human doctors might criticize certain robot brand names, often preferring specific models or systems produced by different companies. Amazingly, some non-medical robots might eventually get involved, publicly "voicing" their own computer-generated concerns.

Retiring Physicians
Human doctors: Stunningly but actually quite possibly, the medical robots might force some people from the profession--the human's positions filled by "mere machines." Limited

percentages of human doctors lucky enough to work until retirement age into their early 60s or 70s will face personal financial catastrohpes, unless they have saved a substantial percentage of their income. This tragedy would worsen on a massive, global human scale if the retiring physicians fail to get the respect that they have earned and richly deserve during their senior years.

   Robots: These machines lack a single "worry" upon their retirement, programmed only to perform their assigned duties-- rather than concentrating on themselves. When deemed no longer useful by society or by the human administrators of facilities where they "worked," a huge percentage of the devices will be sent to scrap yards--to be crushed before their parts are recycled for possible use in future or subsequent robots. These garbage collections would occur regularly on a non-emotional basis, similar to the way used cars are pulverized today.

Example Specifics

   The above examples assume that the robot is an advanced version, built to make its own autonomous decisions and movements. During the initial-transition phase, the earliest prototypes of RoboDocs would merely assist the human doctors; amid that period people ultimately would make any and all vital decisions regarding an individual patient's care. During this phase, chances seem strong that the human doctors will essentially put themselves into a state of "mental denial," always assuming that they could never be replaced by machines. Here is where the human ego comes to play, mirroring a trend that has already occurred for more than a century. Since the late 1800s and early 1900s, machines have consistently and methodically continued to fulfill the tasks once performed by humans. Lots of those instances involved people who initially insisted that machines could never possibly replace them--only to eventually discover otherwise. These many transitions have included: electric lights that replaced the need for whalers for harvesting whale oil; automobiles that replaced the need for stable workers who maintain horses; commercial airliners that decreased demand for passenger trains, forcing many railroad workers to lose their jobs; TV, movies and high-speed Internet, which collectively resulted in a sharp decrease in demand for live amateur stage shows; and many more examples, too numerous to list in full. Keeping these historic examples in mind, if some analysts are to be believed, today's human physicians should stop denying that they will eventually be replaced by machines.

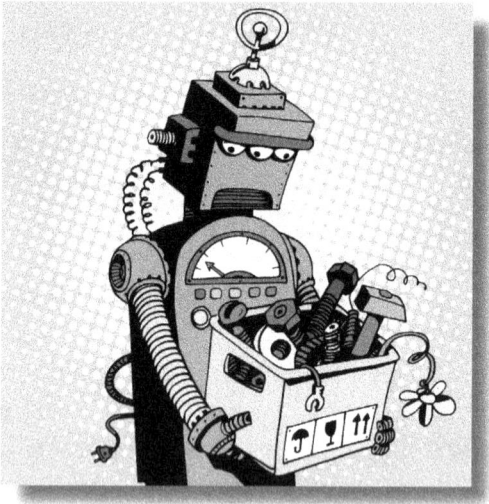

Chapter 17
The Giant Monster ~ Medical Payments

A large, unavoidable monster emerges from the advent of these "spooky" or amazing technologies, mainly: "How will people pay for robotic medical treatments?"

Even before advanced versions of the medical robots get put into full force, this situation already is scary enough to terrify many consumers.

As almost every consumer knows, today's mandatory health insurance systems have already become a catastrophic quagmire for almost everyone involved.

Ultimately this transition comes down to the fact that "if you think that Obamacare is bad, wait until you need to pay for health care involving robots."

To put this travesty into an easily understandable perspective, keep in mind that in the United States health care is a multi-trillion-dollar industry.

Obamacare Serves as a Horrifying Example

Many people rightfully complain that Obamacare is a corrupt, inept and unmanageable system that "attacks consumers, while giving them little or no benefits."

In fact, by some estimates millions of people are now lacking healthcare insurance as a direct result of what I call "Obaminable-care."

The only saving grace in the current situation, at least from the perspective of some people, is that insurance companies can no longer deny coverage to people who suffer from adverse pre-existing medical conditions.

Otherwise, as detailed in two books that I have written about Obamacare, virtually everyone involved suffers due to this ill-conceived law. Those "getting the shaft" include: medical

professionals in almost every health sector; taxpayers in low-
, medium- and high-income brackets; the overall efficiency
and effectiveness of the healthcare industry; and all financially
struggling middle-class families forced to buy expensive policies.

The only people or companies who seem to benefit are the
greedy insurance companies that have a government-authorized
monopoly; and inept politicians who receive massive campaign
contributions from the medical and drug industries.

Government Corruption Accelerates

A whopping 75 percent of Americans agree that the U.S.
government is corrupt, according to a public opinion poll released
by Gallup on September 19, 2015.

Yes, more than ever before everday citizens are convinced
that the U.S. government is "crooked," with three out of every four
people distrusting the federal bureaucracy.

With this factor clearly in focus, the advent of high-
function robots into health care comes at a pivotal time in human
history as most citizens distrust politicians and the federal
government.

A key factor involves massive political campaign
contributions made by wealthy people and major corporations.
Critics insist that our elected leaders are "in the pockets" of
their bigget contributors, resulting in pervasive situations where
politicians continually kowtow to their donors.

Assuming that such allegations are true, do you believe that
politicians and federal bureaucracies always have your best interest
at heart? Do you truly believe that these officials will have your
welfare in mind, when they eventually fine-tune health insurance
regulations in order to accommodate the use of medical robots?

With equal urgency, do you think these decision-makers
will base their choices primarily on "which medical and robotics
companies earns the big money, and how the cash is generated?"

Prepare for a Dire Future

Many of us remember when Congress passed Obamacare in 2010, although the vast majority of Americans surveyed at the time strongly opposed the legislation.

While lots of behind-the-scenes decisions occured, the issue became an intensified focus of debate in open public forums.

Unless Obamacare is scrubbed or retooled, chances seem strong that lots of the vital decisions involving medical robotics will be made behind closed doors.

If that happens as many of us fear, crucial life-and-death decisions involving the robots will occur while the general public is "kept in the dark."

Adding insult to injury, many bureaucrats appointed to Obamacare-related panels have absolutely no medical training. This lame-brained system requires that political appointees or "cronies" make lofty decisions; they decide which medical devices and drugs can be covered by medical insurance--and at what specific price levels.

Will "Political Skulduggery" Endanger You and Your Family?

In all likelihood, many of the most critical questions involving this issue will not get answered or even considered in open public forums.

Meantime, making these hassles even more complex, a related question emerges: "Will all this political skulduggery occur behind the scenes, out of public view?"

Quite disturbingly, if the current crop of politicians is any indication, consumers can expect a worst-case scenraio. This would be the equivalent of immediately before the 2010 passage of Obamacare, when members of Congress had never bothered to read the bill beforehand.

As a prime example, consider the crop of U.S. presidential candidates for election year 2016. On the verge of the first primary caucuses in Iowa, not a single one of these candidates had mentioned robots in-depth or issued any policy statements on this extremely urgent issue--vital to the American culture.

U.S. politicians proved once again that they lack any clue about what is occurring. This disturbing behavior mirrors their consistent overall pattern from the past few hundred years, consistently failing to realize the most critical issues at any given time.

Average Citizens Know More than Politicians

While most or all politicians remained clueless on robotics issues, public opinion surveys showed that average citizens envision significant technological advancements.

According to a Pew Research Survey issued in April 2014, a vast majority of Americans predicted new significant technologies through the mid-2020s.

Besides the advent of drones and robots, many people foresee a world where the vast majority of people have electronic implants in their bodies.

Yes, while politicians remain ignorant about these many potential problems, the general public seems to accept the fact that such changes likely will or can occur.

Worsening matters, some people complain that the government fails to use the best-available technologies to manage or administer federal bureaucracies.

Is "Big Brother" Watching?

Despite the public's general acceptance of advancing technologies in general, many people have limits on what they are willing to tolerate, according to Pew.

The survey indicated that just more than half, or 53 percent, of people indicated that allowing implants of electronic monitoring devices into the human body would be a "change for the worse."

Under some versions of this other-worldly scenario, all people would be required to have medical monitoring devices surgically implanted in their bodies.

Much faster than many people realize, in this futuristic scenario the government would be able to:

Monitor location: Use the global positioning system, or GPS, to continually monitor the position of every living person on earth.

Vital signs: The systems would continully monitor biological vital signs such as body temperature, blood pressure and heart rate--continually sending that data to officials.

Personal actions: Under worst-case scenarios, these machines would continually monitor the person's activities--perhaps even record what has been said.

"Big Brother" Looms

Like this or not, there is no taking away the fact that our government is mega-powerful, capable of invading our personal lives and even dictating healthcare protocols.

This is already happening in the National Security Agency's monitoring of all cell phones, communications and emails on a massive scale.

While all this might seem like an over-the-top scenario that only a paranoid schizophrenic would believe, continual news reports confirm this is occurring.

"Never underestimate the government's potentially devilish intentions," some informed observers might say. "Prepare for the worst, because it likely will occur."

Under this line of thinking the situation "is completely out of your hands," as to the burning question of how to pay for your future robotic medical care--and how much robots will play a role, if at all.

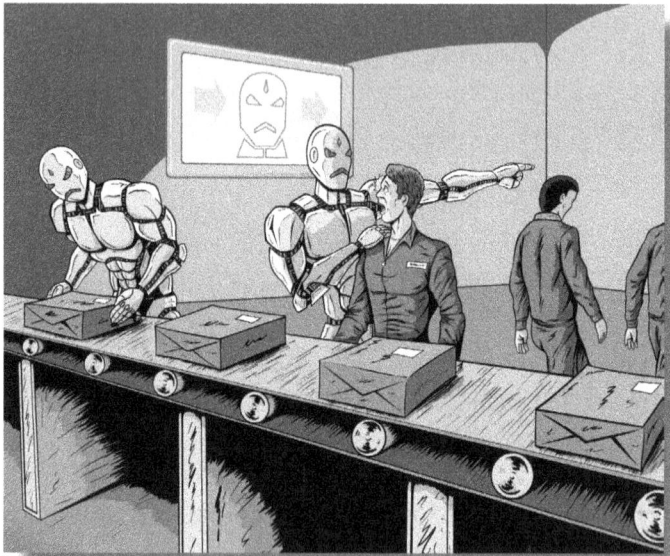

Chapter 18
Beware: The "Rise of the Robots"

The accelerating increase in medical industry machines will occur as robots enter virtually every business sector and society worldwide--on a massive scale.

Yes, consumers will need to adapt their entire lives to the machines, rather than just accommodate for such devices when using the health care industry.

As previously mentioned, increasing numbers of engineers, scientists and economists already are calling this unstoppable trend the "Rise of the Robots." Among just some of these predictions as listed in various 2015 articles in the respected "Business Insider" publication.

2025: A whopping 30 percent of all jobs will be automated due to robotics.

2035: Up to 47 percent of all jobs likely will be taken by robots, according to an Oxford University study reported by "Business Insider."

2040 and beyond: All jobs gradually will be taken by robots, according to predictions by Microsoft founder Bill Gates and physicicist Stephen Hawking.

This Massive Transition has Begun

By late 2015, this massive transition had already clicked into full gear on an international scale, according to various business news reports.

The center of this rapidly spreading trend began in China, where more than 1 million low-skilled workers lost their jobs to robots in a one-year period.

Finding jobs in that nation became a major issue as many millions of additional Chinese people were scheduled to lose their jobs to machines.

The "Bloomberg View" business publication predicted that

80 percent of factory jobs in Guangzhou province would be fully automated by 2020.

Similar transitions were expected to rapidly spread elsewhere, including in the United States where many non-factory jobs are expected to disappear by 2025.

All Job Types Face Elimination

Without exaggeration, virtually every type of job will eventually get targeted for possible elimination, billionaire Bill Gates said during a public forum on the issue.

Besides doctors and other medical professionals, those poised to lose their jobs range form school teachers and police officers to college professors.

"Historically what we thought was that robots would do things that were the three D's--dangerous, dirty and dull," Ryan Calo, a robotics expert and professor at University of Washington School of Law told "Business Insider." "Over time, the range of things that robots can do has extended."

In fact, the advancements in robotics are going so fast, according to Ray Kurzweil, Google's director of engineering, that by 2029 robots will surpass the intelligence of humans. This obviously puts a big fear in doctors and other professionals who insist that "my job could never be taken by a mere machine."

Yet the robotics industry already was charging full speed ahead by the mid-2010s, when electrical engineers announced major advancements on a daily basis.

Media and Government Remained "Oblivious"

Shockingly, the mainstream news media and politicians as an overall group remained "fully in the dark, oblivious to this growing issue."

For the most part newspapers, TV programs and radio reports treated these groundbreaking stories as mere novelties-- delegated to the "quirky news."

A casual observer might incorrectly think that this was "no big deal."

To the contrary, however, the overall transition was far more "real" than many imagined. Among just some of the many initial transitions destined to become major milestones:

Store greeters: Increasing numbers of department stores in Asia, especially Japan, started using robots rather than people to greet shoppers as they entered the businesses.

Newscaster: Lifelike, news-reading robots began appearing on Japanese TV.

Police officers: By mid-2015, robots began serving as police officers in Dubai.

"People need to get ready, because these changes seem unstoppable," a close observer might say. "Almost every aspect of our lives is destined to change in a drastic way, a significant transition forcing each person to adapt."

Notice the "Big Picture"

Whether they want to or not, people needing the healthcare industry after 2025 will encounter far more robots than the merely devices used at hospitals and clinics.

Gradually over the next few decades robots will play significant roles in all of our lives, from the moment we awaken each morning--clear until bedtime.

Even while we're asleep, if engineers and scientists are successful in their ongoing efforts, robotic machines will continually monitor our vital signs.

Yes, the so-called "big brother" is on the way, the machines now under development by universities, corporations and the world's most powerful governments.

People who today consider themselves as "far from tech-savvy," will need or want to learn ways to interact with these increasingly advanced machines.

Learn Vital Basics About Robots

By this point anyone discovering the advent of medical machines for the first time should appreciate the urgent need to understand basics of the Rise of the Robots.

As you might imagine, this overall complex puzzle has many interacting parts and issues. So, in subsequent chapters you will learn much more, including:

Interaction: How will these wide-scale transitions interact with and impact general industry in many business sectors, rather than just the robots designed for hospitals and clinics?

Robotics: What is the history and concept of robots, and how will that impact your life and those of your loved ones?

Designers: Who is building and designing the machines, while envisioning and creating new technoligies necessary for these transitions?

Specific Technologies: How will specific new robotic technologies impact, help or potentially harm specific healthcare specialties?

The World's Largest Growth Industry

In-depth, science-based and broad-scale business forecasts involving the impact of robots on all of society are difficult--if not impossible--to find.

Even so, robotics could easily surge into the biggest growth industry in human history, at least judging by the forecasts of scientists and economists.

If advancements continue as expected, dominance by the robotics industry seems quite plausible; massive growth seems probable in this business sector, particularly as the machines play an seemingly irreplaceable role throughout society.

Sadly, if even some of these predictions prove correct, from the perspective of many people "the heart of humanity" will become overly dependent on robots.

Some scientists including internationally acclaimed

physicist Stephen Hawking worry that these machines will eventually dominate and control all people; under this scenario humans would become an endangered species--or even extinct.

According to various news reports, at an accelerated pace from 2012 to 2015, scientists had already created systems and technologies that enabled robots to build similar machines at a rapid-fire pace.

More than Merely Science Fiction

Collectively and individually, these transitions impress many people as being "mere science fiction, just a wild, impossible fantasy that never will or could occur."

To the contrary, however, judging from news reports and scientific papers these transitions are well underway--in many instances to the point of being unstoppable.

At least from the view of many people, the most horrifying examples involve military robots. (These are worthy of a subsequent chapter.)

Upon learning about these advancements in all business sectors for the first time, many people understandably become fearful or timid about the future.

Adding more reason for "future shock," many of these technologies are progressing so fast that average people realize that they will remain helpless to stop these horrifying transitions.

Put Everything into Clear Perspective

As individuals, families and as a society we have an urgent need to identify and to understand the many robot-caused changes. Among the actual films available for free viewing on the Internet are images that "drive home the fact that these efforts are real:"

Teachers: In various countries worldwide, robots are shown in classrooms, teaching eager students at elementary schools and even higher levels of eduction. So, will millions of teachers will lose their jobs to robots? Some people fear this will occur if heartless governments and school districts strive to eliminate any need to pay teachers.

Police officers: Briefly mentioned earlier, could this transition grow to the point where human "peace officers" are eliminated from the equation? As shocking as this might seem, could "RoboCops" eventually arrest you, kill you or even enslave you or your family? Well, like this or not, robotic police officers are already being designed and put into service, initially on a limited basis.

Military robots: Steadily increasing numbers of short films and educational documentaries feature disturbing images of seemingly indestructable military robots. Under worst-case scenarios, if development goes as planned, could these machines be capable of conquering entire countries--killing every person "at will?"

The handful of crucial examples already described here comprise only a tiny portion of the many potential significant uses for robots in the near future.

Life-Saving Service Robots

One of the most admirable and useful goals of electrical engineers and scientists focuses on the development of robots that would save the lives of public safety personnel.

The positive side of this sector involves the creation of robots that would serve as firefighters and--as previously mentioned--police officers and soldiers.

Under such a system, the "mere machines" would go into harm's way--eliminating the need for people to risk severe injury or death. A possble ripple effect might result, decreasing the number of people needing intensive medical care.

Yet on the flip-side, many millions of public service personnel might eventually become jobless. Unless people are successful in blocking this transition, the complete change would occur at the point when robots become highly advanced.

Additional "shock value" comes to play when realizing that the robotic cops and military robots would be able to quickly and easily inflict people with horrific injuries or kill them.

Under so-called best-case scenarios, initial prototypes or early versions of these robots would start by working alongside people; then, subsequent highly advanced updates of the machines would replace the humans.

The medical industry likely would experience similar transitions, with earlier versions of robots initially assisting human medical professionals, before the machines eventually replace healthcare professionals.

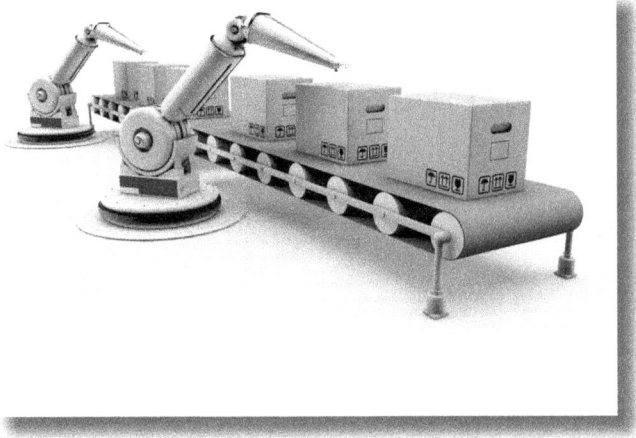

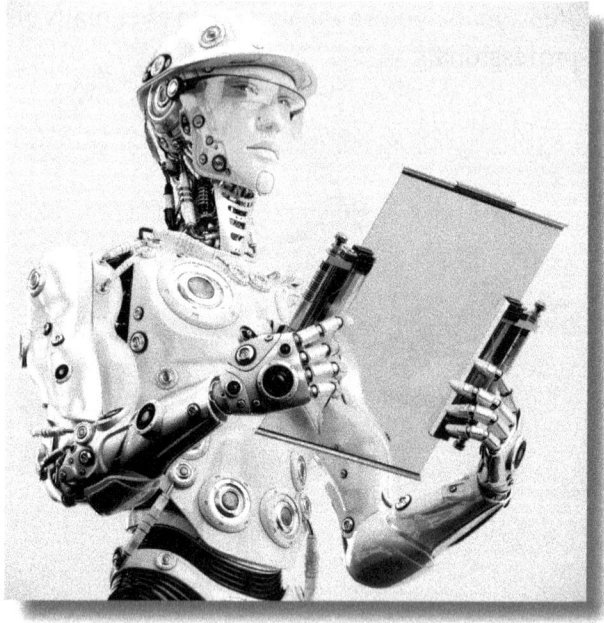

Chapter 19
Employment Issue Swells ~ Robots "Steal" Our Jobs

Besides the potential for endangering public health, the biggest issue by far stemming from the Rise of Robots will involve millions of people losing their jobs.

Keep in mind the aforementioned fact that tens of millions or perhaps even billions of people will become unemployed within the next few decades if robots spread into society as some experts predict.

Could this evolve into one of humanity's worst tragedies, far more destructive than previous world-changing events such as deadly plagues that killed many millions of people from the 1300s through the 1600s?

The Black Death plague that killed an estimated 70 million to 200 million people, starting in 1346, took nearly 400 years for mankind to understand and control. By comparison, potential health problems stemming from killer or military robots might become impossible to control.

In summary, humanity faces adverse changes unless officials take decisive action soon to ensure that more good than harm comes from the Rise of the Robots.

Society's Biggest Challenge

As briefly mentioned earlier, many people have lost their jobs due to technological advances since the late 1800s. Yet those changes impacting specific industries never occurred simultaneously worldwide in all industries.

By comparison, society's ability to adequately cope with the Rise of Robots in the employment arena seems dismal. Among the many specific reasons:

Politicians: Consistently mentioned here as a key part of society's problems, our elected leaders have done nothing

143

significant to develop solutions that would enable society to cope with or benefit from robotics.

Businesses: The many businesses and industry sectors quietly striving to advance robotics have failed to announce efforts to re-train or help people who lose their jobs.

Regulation: The world's largest governments, particularly the United States, seem to lack sufficient regulations to keep robots from "getting out of control."

Difficult Challenge

Envision a world where only half of all adults have jobs, and then eventually almost every person lacks employment or a source of income.

How would these people earn adequate funds for life-sustaining food, clothing and shelter?

For now, there are no reliable answers. Perhaps just as disturbing, would humanity manage to develop a system where everyone receives life's basic necessities for "free"--because robots have robbed people of an ability to earn?

With equal urgency, how such a governmental infrastructure would work or even get implemented remains a huge uncertainty.

Ultimately, we all must face the fact that no one at this juncture can predict precisely how society and health care will evolve.

The late president John Fitzgerald Kennedy, assassinated in 1963, proclaimed in his inauguration speech that "God's work on this earth must truely be our own."

Assuming that is correct, are advanced robots "ungodly and inhumane?" What justifies attempts to create machines to do "God's work on earth?"

Like this or not, these are questions that society as a whole will be forced by circumstances to answer--that is, assuming that enough time remains to regulate or control the Rise of the Robots.

Robotics Endanger More than Jobs

Far more than merely concentrating on the employment issue, a second joint statement in 2015 by Stephen Hawking, business leaders and scientists warned against government efforts to develop autonomous weapons that use AI--machines capable of making their own decisions amid war.

"If any military power pushes ahead with AI weapon development, a global arms race is vitrually inevitable," the statement said. "And, the endpoint of this technology trajectory is obvious: autonomous weapons will become the Kalashnikovs of tomorrow.

"Unlike nuclear weapons, they contain no costly or hard-to-obtain raw materials, so they will become ubiquitous and cheap for all significant military powers to mass-produce.

"It will only be a matter of time before they appear on the black market and in the hands of terrorists, dictators wishing to better control their populace, warlords wishing to perpetuate ethnic cleansing, etc.

"Autonomous weapons are ideal for tasks such as assassinations, destabilizing nations, subduing populations and selectively killing a particular ethnic group."

Chaotic Situation Generates Mass Confusion

As if robotic weaponary wasn't already enough of a concern, while the "robots-and-jobs" issue intensified in October 2015, the news media issued conflicting stories on the impact that these advanced machines will have on employment.

"Robots have transformed the lives of tradesmen and laborers, but lawyers, architects and doctors tend to believe that their careers are safe from the advances of Artificial Intelligence," said an Oct. 14, 2015 story at the "QZ" news Website. This belief is "entirely wrong," according to the upcoming book, 'Future of the Professions: How Technology Will Transform the Work of Human Experts.'"

According to the "QZ" story, the authors--a visiting professor at Oxford Internet Institute, Richard Susskind, and his son, a lecturer at the same institution--conducted 100 interviews--while drawing on economic and sociological theory.

"QZ" said the Susskinds concluded, that "AI will dramatically transform the middle-class working landscape."

In the near-term, the Susskinds argue, Artificial Intelligence "will simply accelerate the efficiency of professions. But then robots will start to take over more work, and the humans will find the roles of 'doctor' or 'lawyer' replaced with less glamorous-sounding titles as 'emphathizer,' 'knowledge engineer,' or 'system provider.'"

The authors' in-depth analysis concludes that only the "very top" human professionls will retain work--with the best and brightest enduring the longest, while "armies of professionals" fail to maintain or to get gainful employment.

Vastly Differing Opinions Emerged

Giving a vastly different approach, just three days after the "QZ" report, in "Forbes" economics and finance section, writer Tim Worstall--a contributor on economics, finance and public policy--downplayed the potential job-loss dangers caused by robotics.

Worstall's opinion becomes clear right away in the headline: "Don't Fear the Robots Stealing Our Jobs: The Labor Department Tells Us Why."

"The message from this report is that we really don't need to fear the robots coming to steal all our jobs," Worstall said. "You know, that version where they do all the work and we do all the consuming. Or is it the version where they do all the work and we starve, as we've got no way of earning anything? The real question here is in fact at what speed this might happen."

Worstall goes on to argue that everything hinges on whether people get to consume what robots produce. In essence, he insists that robots will do absolutely nothing to change the economy unless people are able to generate enough income to consume or "buy" things.

Under this argument, the building of robots would not make economic sense for producers of the machines, unless there are enough people or corporations in society with sufficient incomes to purchase and benefit from the devices.

Growth in Certain Professions Forecast

Amid the increasingly intense issue regarding who is most likely to lose their jobs, experts list numerous courses or majors that college students should take to drastically improve their employment prospects:

Microbiotics and genomics: Those with a keen understanding of living cells position themselves for jobs at companies that develop medical robotics or any type of machine designed to manipulate DNA or cell structures.

Mathematics and physics: Robotics is essentially a "numbers game," dependant on intrinsic calculations necessary for developing machines that work at maximum capacity. These factors regulate the design and manufacturing of robot parts.

Logistical studies: Some universities offer high-level courses in logistics, which is the business, process and science of efficiently getting information and materials together. Collectively and individually, these interlinked factors are necessary for the manufacturing and delivery of cost-effective and profitable products and services. When performed at optimal levels, the "logistics process" enables the creation, production and distribution of goods and services--in this case made possible by robotics.

Information technology: Nicknamed "IT," these students learn the intricacies of efficiently storing, protecting, sharing and distributing information--usually on Web-based platforms. Advanced robots will depend on high-level IT, particularly for the instant analysis and calculations of information.

Chemistry and metallurgy: Students learning the

intricacies of these sciences might position themselves for jobs necessary in the building and designing of durable robots. Such skills and parts are necessary for building viable or long-lasting machines.

Electrical engineering: Along with structural engineering, professionals with these advanced high-level college degrees concentrate on the actual creation and building of robots and other high-level machines.

Ultimately, skilled human administrators and managers will be necessary for coordinating all of the various above-listed skills and technologies--at least to the point when robots theoretically assume those duties. In best-case scenarios, the designing and building of high-level robots involves efficient one-on-one work with various robotics-creation team leaders and managers.

Another Dire Forecast: University Closures

The overall future of robotics and the need for humans to remain an integral part of this process becomes even more dire, particularly when considering the dismal forecasts about the future of universities and colleges worldwide.

Specificis of these gloomy predictions seem to depend on who makes the forecasts and how.

Yet there seems to be widespread agreement that lots of these institutions will close at an accelerating pace.

On Sept. 28, 2015, in a story for "Inside Higher Ed," Kellie Woodhouse described a Moody's Investor Service prediction that the closures of small colleges and universities would triple in the next several years--while mergers of such institutions double.

On average during the previous decade, about five of these institutions closed every year. But according to Moody's, the total was expected to triple by 2017.

Will Robots Reduce the Need for Universities?

At a steadily increasing rate through 2015, disturbing news emerged detailing analysts' predictions that university closures would accelerate.

"I don't think it's going to be a landslide of college closures, but it's going to be a very rough period of time," senior Moody's vice president Susan Fitzgerald said, quoted in a March 28, 2015, "Market Watch" story.

Rather than robots or automated employment systems, these initial closures of the institutions were caused by decreasing revenues--amid enrollment declines.

University administrators refrained from saying so, but could future job losses caused by robots worsen the problem facing universities and colleges?

Well, if the forecasts of a steady rise in robotics occurs as expected, a sharp and negative impact on higher eductation seems possible or even probable.

Why Attend Universities if Robots Take Most Jobs?

Shockingly, the need for universities and higher education courses would shrink and eventually disappear, if the scenario mentioned by Stephen Hawking comes true.

"Why in the world would I want to attend to college?" some prospective students might proclaim. "There is no sense to learn, if there are an extremely limited number of jobs, or no employment whatsoever."

The average undergraduate degree costs well over $100,000, and in some instances much more. Many students or their families go into extensive debt to make their dreams of a better life come true, thanks to the benefits of higher education.

With luck, hopefully society's widespread transition into a "robot culture" will occur at a slow, steady pace--rather than a rapid-fire rate. Otherwise, imagine the financial catastrophe facing students and society as a whole.

"The overall dilemma and the proverbial 'steamroller of technology' have gotten so massive, this critical situation is getting much too large," some people might complain. "The average person will be able to do little or nothing to stop this situation."

Negative "Ripple Effect" Throughout Society

Would rapidly accelerating university closures amid the Rise of the Robots generate a disastrous worldwide conomic impact?

Such a catastrophe would devastate the United States, where most large cities nationwide are "university towns." Comprising a huge chunk of the U.S. economy, these communities serve as the backbone for business and industry.

Closures of the institutions would force extensive operational cutbacks at many thousands of small and large businesses, resulting in countless job losses.

Cognizant of these critial factors, an essential question emerges: "Have the worst widespread university closures already begun?"

This seems plausible. After all, high school graduation rates decreased or flattened nationwide by early 2015, forcing the number of potential college students to stagnate.

In March of that year, the University of Phoenix announced that its student levels had declined by half since 2010. The downturn forced the institution to close more than 100 of its campuses nationwide, according to a March 2015 story by "CNN Money."

Impact on Medical Schools

The potential impact of this disturbing trend on medical schools and on pre-med undergraduate programs apparently remained unknown.

A sharp downturn in enrollment, or closures of those institutions, would generate a widespread negative economic impact. The heatlhcare industry's educational, research and instructional expenses are much higher than most business sectors.

Precisely how this will play out remains a pivotal factor. At this early juncture, officials seem to ack any precise estimates on how university closures or consolidations would impact medical schools.

Even without this necessary data, as more prospective doctors and lawyers experience a downturn in their industries, why would potential students--who might otherwise hope to enter those professions--even want to attend?

For most medical and law students during the past few centuries, attending such institutions has always been a proverbial "roll of the dice." Through many generations, only a handful of such students have been guaranteed jobs well before or even after graduation.

Even so, most of these students until now have known that they had a fairly good chance of landing good jobs. Such certainty likely will disappear due to the Rise of the Robots, coupled with ongoing challenges facing higher education.

Caught in a Big Squeeze

Those experiencing the most difficulties in this arena might include professors or instructors without tenure, and students who enter university or college programs just as the robotic transition finally starts "clicking into full gear."

When they finally graduate, following years of study and high expense, these students might eventually learn to their great disappointment that the potentially lucrative jobs they studied for no longer exist.

In a classic "domino effect," such scenarios would--in turn--lead to a sharp decrease in enrollments or even more university closures. Tragically, as a result many non-tenured professors and teaching assistants would become unemployed.

Worsening the situation, under this scenario the students would be "left holding the bag," saddled with huge tuition debt--without the necessary current or future income to pay off their college debts.

At present, this situation is either a catastrophic avalanche waiting to happen, or authorities will somehow miraculously prevent such an outcome.

Right now potential university students who have just

graduated from high school could find themselves locked into an inescapable dilemma. Yet at least some hope remains, particulary among those who qualify for--and who choose--to concentrate their studies on subjects leading to viable professions that are the most likely to survive the Rise of the Robots.

Problems Faced by Newborns

Every child born in the United States in 2015 and beyond will face the biggest employment challenges due to the projected advancements in robotics.

Indeed, chances of getting a good, high-paying job when they finally reach their adult years would seem insurmountable or even infinitesimal.

Or, is such a statement a wild exaggeration, intended to instill unnecessary and unwarranted fear throughout society?

Well, if the so-called experts are to be believed, the projected advancements in robotics seem to be a certainty--particularly within the health care industry.

"Children born after 2020 will have little chance of ever getting gainful employment," some people might complain. "What need is there to attend school in a robot-dominated society where people seemingly have a better chance of winning a lottery than landing a good job?"

Chapter 20
Brain Microchips

Many people fail to realize this, but scientists already are developing and implanting microchips into the brains of animals--including people.

In the long-term, researchers hope that this process will generate technology that enables humans to benefit from instant access to massive amounts of information.

Imagine merely thinking of a specific topic, and then instantly getting access to all related information at little or no cost--instantly sent into the human brain. Ideally, such a system would be manageable and beneficial, enhancing the person's lifestyle, while increasing the individual's efficiency.

Naturally, to most people discovering this concept for the first time, such a system seems like "just a bunch of fantasy." After all, any rational person today would think that such a system would only become possible thousands of years from now--if at all.

Yet today's real-world scientists claim that they already are developing such systems. In fact, early prototypes of computer-based microchips already are being implanted into the brains of U.S. soldiers who suffered critical head injuries in battle.

Medical Industry Impact

Brain microchips would significantly impact all industries, particularly health care. However, the potential impact remains a "big unknown," on how these technological advances will impact society, families, mankind's overall quality of life, the economy and business in general.

Would the advent of such a system rapidly accelerate university closures? Just as perplexing, will brain microchips eventually make low-IQ people suddenly behave much smarter--putting them on par with people naturally blessed with vastly superior intelligence than most other individuals?

From the view of educational institutions and scientists, the demand for such technology could easily reach extraordinary levels. Yet, why would anyone want or permit surgeons to install such devices into their bodies?

Envisioning such situations might seem like a mere guessing game at this point. Yet the motivations of most people getting them might seem obvious.

First, lots of people using such devices would want to remain competitive with other humans throughout society. Under this line of thinking, "why would you want to walk around behaving like a typical dummy, while everyone else using the devices automatically has vastly superior survival skills and also essentially keeps you in your place as an inferior?"

Then there is the added concern that people using brain microchips will have a greater ability to complete for jobs, food, money, and desired relationships.

Technological Advancements Have Made this Possible

The technology needed for brain microchips has been made possible by significant advancements in the understanding of genomics and the human brain, according to the U.S. government's Defense Advanced Research Projects Agency-- sometimes called "DARPA."

Interestingly, this is the same federal bureaucracy assigned to monitor and help coordinate the concepts, design and development of highly destructive military robots.

A Sept. 28, 2015, article by Mary-Ann Russon for "International Business Times," describes a book revealing that DARPA is already implanting microchips into the brains of soldiers wounded in Iraq and Afghanistan.

Russon's article said that officials launched the effort as part of President Barack Obama's August 2014 directive, ordering that the government develop technology to improve the mental health of soldiers and veterans.

"One of the plans included developing computer chips

that could be implanted within the brain's tissue to help regulate the nervous system," the story said. This process "would help to alleviate symptoms of a variety of conditions from post-traumatic stress disorder (PTSD) to arthritis."

Technology Rapidly Accelerated

The initial leap into this new realm occurred in 2012, when the "IO9" service reported that for the first time scientists had used microchips to increase the intelligence of monkeys.

"Scientists have demonstrated that a brain implant can improve thinking ability in primates," the "IO9" report said. "By implanting an electrode array into the celebral cortex of monkeys, researchers were able to restore--and even improve--their (the animals') decision-making abilities.

"The implication for possible therapies are far-reaching, including potential treatments for cognitive disorders and brain injuries."

Since then, this has become possible at greater levels because scientists, working in cooperation with biologists and doctors, have accurately mapped the brains of primates.

These tasks have been monumental, largely because the brain has many billions of individual neurons, according to an October 2015 report in "Lab News."

Disturbing Discoveries Continue

Such landmark discoveries have progressed at a rapid rate unseen in any other industry, according to a report by Ed John in the "Mancunion," a publication from the Manchester Media Group.

"Whether it be for the social, economic or medicinal aspects of our lives, it is undeniable that we are rapidly heading for an existence in which we are rarely detached from technology's influence," John said. "Whilst this growth has its indisputable benefits, are we really ready for the world which we seem so desperate to attain?"

John is among a growing number of analysts or observers who worry that such advancements are undermining--or will degrade--the basic experience of being human.

They argue that the development and use of such technologies have been a fantasy for people for a long time. Yet as a result of mankind's relentless and non-stop research, testing and robotics creations, such systems are "becoming reality;" this leaves some researchers and scientists "literally stunned" by what they have actually designed and built.

Benefitting from the scientists' discoveries in brain-microchip technologies, increasing numbers of U.S. military veterans who suffered head injuries now have brain microchips. Amazingly, these devices enable some of these former soldiers to use their brains to move the previously mentioned robotic limbs.

Diverse Microchip Implants Developed

Most undergoing continual modifications for design improvements, with varying degrees of success the various future microchip implants would include:

Diabetes: Microchips implanted inside the forearms of diabetics. The devices continually monitor blood sugar, immediately notifying the person to eat certain foods, take medications, or inject insulin.

Data: Briefly mentioned earlier, certain microchips would enable living brains to receive "inhuman amounts of data." If successful, this could change humanity forever.

Vital signs: Specialized implanted microchips would continually monitor all primary biological vital signs including heart rate, body temperature, blood pressure, and breathing. This would enable doctors to continually monitor patient health.

Personal Monitoring: These devices, likely to become highly controversial when the general public finally learns about them, would continually monitor the person's location throughout his or her lifetime. Critics likely will complain about a loss of personal freedoms.

Communications: According to numerous news reports, scientists keep striving to design functional and reliable brain microchips that will allow people to continually communicate with individuals who have similar implants. This would happen without cell phones or computers.

Medical Implications Have Tremendous Potential

As an overall sector, microchip implants seem to present a tremendous potential for benefitting the entire health care industry--but only if done "the right way."

Scientists and particuarly doctors who assist them need to use extreme caution when designing and creating microchip implants.

By going too far, striving to overachieve much more than necessary, robotics engineers might develop "gimmickry" unhealthful for humanity.

Imagine a world where microchips have been implanted into most or even all vital organs of every living person.

From the perspective of humanity, what we experience alone or collectively as humans would change forevermore. Within such a warped society, full-bodied and natural people would no longer exist.

Such possibilities, in turn, bring up a crucial question that will override all of humanity for as long people remain alive: "Especially among those who believe in a loving and giving God, what right have we as mere humans to tinker with, change or modify what our Creator has lovingly made for us all--our natural bodies?"

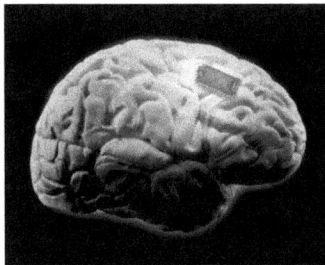

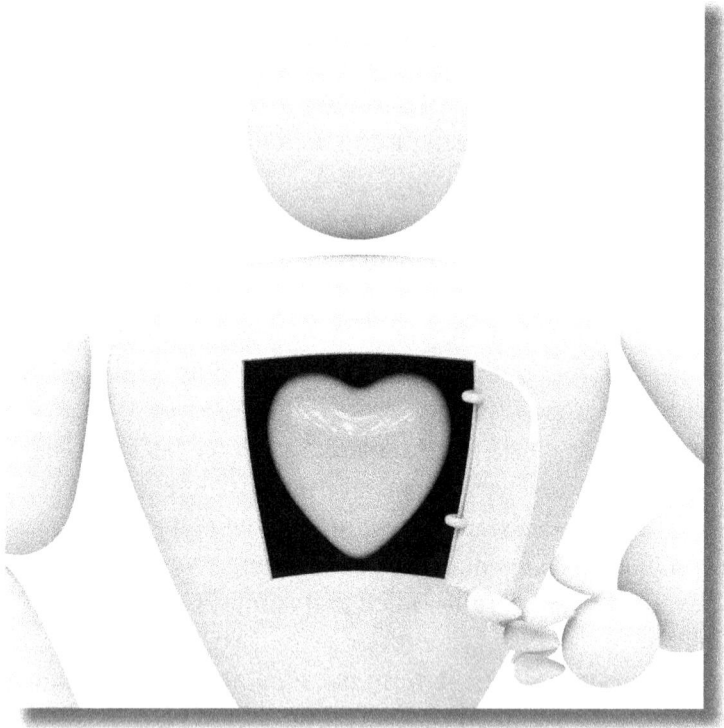

Chapter 21
Sex With Robots Becomes Controversial

Even during the second decade of the 21st Century, some people who took the time to follow these issues label the trend as "disturbing" or even "immoral."

Sometimes mentioned as an excellent example is the RealDoll (tm), a robot designed to have sex with humans. At the request of this machine's producer, electrical engineers have been developing robotic characteristics similar to people having sex.

The effort has drawn criticisms and even jokes. Yet overall such programs are considerd a serious endeavor, with some sociologists going so far as to project that by 2050 human beings will be having more sex with machines than with people.

Dubbed "RoboSex," such encounters could evolve into a full-fledged, multi-trillion-dollar industry. While generating mountains of cash this way might sound intriguing; the mere thought of sexual interaction between machines and humans strikes some people as repulsive, inhuman and even "against the will of God."

The hottest issue here centers on the obliteration of human-to-human relationships, in many ways the "very core and essence of what it means to be a person."

Scientists, doctors and biologists have known for many generations that besides hunger and an innate desire for shelter, the innate, natural and continual drive for sex hails as perhaps the most powerful, natural and instinctive human motivations.

Will RoboSex Destroy Humanity?

From the view of critics, a society that allows or encourages people to have sex with robots could wreak havoc on the very essence of "what it means to be human."

The Internet is already loaded with videos and films of early prototypes of sexual robots. These machines often become "big hits" at various robotics or sex industry conventions. Some videos feature humans behaving as if surprised that they actually get "turned on" while looking that these machines--some devices wearing skimpy undergarments.

Despite such cheers and laughter, however, such machines spark sharp criticism for a variety of legitimate reasons. Among them:

Resolving conflicts: Human beings naturally strive to resolve or "fix" their human-to-human relationship problems with their chosen mates or sex partners. Depending on the specific circumstances, people often need to modify their own behaviors in order to accommodate the desires or demands of their "focus of sexual desire"--in order to eventually enjoy, and hopefully engage in, consensual physical intimacy. For instance, although this might seem like a laughing matter to some, a husband who dislikes taking out the garbage will often do so anyway to keep his wife in a calm and peaceful mood necessary to among other factors to put here in the mood for--or make willing to engage in--sex.

Purchase preferences: A husband who is sick and tired of taking out the garbage in order to put his wife in the mood might buy a "female" robot that never nags about such things. As a prime example, a human husband in his 60s might choose to buy a feminine RoboSex machine with all the physicial characteristics he prefers: big firm boobs; tight waist; nice round and firm posterior; long and flowing blonde hair; and magnetic blue eyes--all characteristics that his human wife lacks. Just as essential from the man's view in this hypothetical instance, the guy also could choose a robot that only says nice, sexy things to him--never bringing up family issues, needing "romance," or nagging him to do chores.

Shunning other humans: When"perfect" robots become available for companionship and sex, why would any human ever want or need to have a relationship with an imperfect person? Just imagine having an ideal "love bond," getting the perfect "artificial person"--a made-to-order humanoid that fulfills your every desire.

If desired, you would never have to adapt to the needs, wishes and demands of other people. Yet instead of searching for a person with such attributes, you could buy a "dfficult robot" that has these challenging personality characteristics. As a result, thoughout any society where humanoid sex robots thrive, any real-live, fulfilling and complex person-to-person relationships would become rare or non-existent.

Shocking Outcome

Perhaps most disturbing, at least from the view of people eager to save humanity, in a society filled with human-like sex robots, the birth rate of actual humans theoretically could plummet to critically low levels or even zero. These overriding fears grip the emotions of some people who study this issue.

Among the many disturbing potential outcomes likely to impact the healthcare industry:

Robo Marriage: Mirroring the "gay marriage" human rights effort of the 2010 to 2015, by the mid-2030s and beyond people "in love" with robots likely will launch intense political campaigns for legally binding robot-and-human marriage rights. At least this is the trend envisioned by some sociologists. According to the "Daily Mail," the first official nuptials involving robots occurred when two machines married each other in Japan. The headline proclaimed, "The Bride Wore White, and the Groom Wore Out His Batteries." Will this emerging trend blossom on an international scale?

Legal Obligations: As bizarre as this might seem, it's true--lawmakers and courts might have to wrangle with complex legal issues. Among the key questions: Will the possessions of people who "marry" robots be legally bounded or co-owned by the machines? For instance, many states including Nevada and California enforce "community property" laws--where each of the two married people share a 50-percent ownership of cash and property. After a "married" robot irreparably breaks or a person dies, will human heirs legally fight for a greater share of inheritance--their legal adversaries being "robotic offspring" produced in factories?

Homicide: Assuming that advanced humanoids become top-notch and human-like, would destroying one of the machines the legal equivalent of "murder." Or, would such a crime be categorized as the equivalent of stealing a car? If a person marries a robot and then that machine gets destroyed by another person, the widow or widower might consider such a crime to be "nothing less than murder."

Mental Health: Some people likely will suffer extreme mental health issues, falling just as much in "love" with a particular robot as the humans would with a person. Unlike people though, an "individual robot" might be fully replaceable--identical in every way to a new robot. This might mean that the robot theoretically would be able to "live forever," while the human lifespan remains extremely limited, to perhaps a 105-year maximum--at least until the point when scientists develop technology that enables individual persons to live for hundreds, or even thousands of years. This way the person never would have to endure the emotional heartache of losing their most beloved robot to death. Yet some observers might argue that the natural end-of-life process is actually a "good thing." Since the earliest people long ago, permanent loss such as death has forced survivors to learn how to cope and endure through emotional pain. This is a sharp contrast to a society where people permanently marry and bond with indestructable robots.

Questioning Morality

Many people might argue that intimate machine-and-person relationships are "sinful," because God created humans as superior creatures on this earth--each with a soul.

Adding to the complexity to this issue, other humans or even robots might insist that machines are just as important to the universe. This is likely to strike many of them as logical because all physical objects in the universe including people and machines are comprised of the same materials--everything from metals to gasses, chemicals and basic elements.

Devout Christians such as myself would dispute such a notion on moral and religious grounds. I fully believe in my heart, mind and soul that people have a God-given superiority to other animals and inanimate objects in the universe. Any contention that robots are the equivalent to humans should be considered "immoral and against the will of God."

However, lots of people are likely to insist otherwise. These humans are likely to eventually petition the courts and lobby lawmakers, in much the same way that gay people did in championing their legal right to marry each other.

By forecasting such a trend, I am in no way trying to imply that gay humans are the legal and moral equivalent of robots. From my view, to even imply that would be sinful as well because--as I have already indicted--I consider humans to be superior to machines.

Challenging Medical Issues

The relationships between robots and humans likely will have a profound impact on the medical industry. Consumers should expect multiple phases in this regard:

Transition period: While human doctors continue "working," and for as long as as robots continue to assist them, physicians likely will need to communicate with their human patients--and also with their relatives or spouses, some of whom are actually robots. Needless to say, the mere thought of such a dilemma seems ludicrous at this point. But those of us "unbelievers" in robotics would need to adapt in a mental and psychological sense, bowing to the supposed need to talk with "robotic relatives."

Profound change: At the point where RoboDocs fully replace human physicians, all communication between machine doctors would be automatic--via Web-based wi fi hookups. A unique mix of "strange" and "tragedy" emerges, with humans literally wiped out of the decision-making process--at least in instances where the patient goes into a coma, and the individual's only living "relatives" are machines.

Pulling the Plug: Well into the 2010s, patients in many hospitals were able to compose or authorize legally-acceptable "end-of-life documents." These are essentially last wills and testaments, at least in a medical sense; the documents specify when, if and how doctors should "pull the plug" on life support systems when the person enters a vegitative state. Now, in cases where a patient enters such a catastrophic and irreversable physical condition, the patient's human relatives must decide whether to stop life-support systems. Later, when and if robots start marrying people as some experts predict, authorities would need to consider enacting or outlawing "robot-relatives" from making life-and-death decisions for people.

Analysts Make Serious Observations

In her critique of David Harper's 2007 book, "Love + Sex With Robots: The Evolution of Human-Robot Relationships," Rachel Maines, a visiting scholar at Cornell University, admits she had a positive reaction to the publication.

Writing for "Research Gate," Maines described the book as a "provocative and engaging romp through the prediction that by the middle of this century robots will have joined the extended human family that now includes dogs, cats, horses, and their virtual counterparts, and will have taken on the characteristics that in the old feminist joke, induced God to create men: She realized that vibrators couldn't dance. When robots dance, make eye contact, smile, make jokes and simulate love for us, I find it entirely plausible that some of us will love them in return."

Taking a much less whimsical approach, Eleanor Robertson wrote a 2014 review in "The Guardian" of the groundbreaking movie "Her," starring Juaquin Phoenix. The film explores the strong emotional attachment and love between a man, Theodore, played by Phoenix and Samantha, a female robot in cyberspace. The virtual robot is ideally suited for his personality.

"The film's aesthetic is gauzy, priming you to go 'aww' in much the same way as a nappy commercial, and the characters communicate largely through trite emotional remarks that wouldn't be out of place in one of the teeth-achingly mawkish love letters Theodore writes for a living," Robertson's review says. "The upshot of this sickly sweet tone is that the audience is directed to look through a Vaseline-covered lens at the film's actual plot, which runs along the lines of 'emotionally stunted man-child conducts unethical dalliance with robot housemaid, (and) learns some serious lessons about himself.'"

On the downside, reviews, observations and films such as these do little--if anything--to describe and convey the many critical issues that humans are likely to face when emotionally attached to robots. Yet at least society as a whole is acknowledging the steadily inceasing complexity of this emerging issue, the imprecise and difficult-to-describe interactions between people and machines.

Trust Issue Flares Up

In her 2013 article for "Live Science," entitled "Human-Robot Relations: Why We Should Worry," Clara Moskowitz urges people to carefully examine their relationship with machines "before it's too late."

Moskowitz quoted an expert who argued that even by then machines already were beginning to disrupt or block interactions among people.

She quoted a professor of social studies and science at Massachusetts Institute of Technology, Sherry Turkle, who insists that instead of interacting with other humans, some people are getting companionship from various toys and electronic tools.

These included Apple's iPhone digital assistant called "Siri," plus any technology that enables humans to find, learn and rely on new machines. Although not highly advanced robots, such innovations already are impacting humans well before high-

165

functioning machines enter the marketplace. Eventually, the article says, advanced robots are envisioned as future teachers for the young and companions for seniors.

"The idea of some kind of artificial companionship has already become the new normal," the article quoted Turkle as saying. "Kids play with robotic pets, (and) become allies with computer game agents. But I think that this new normal comes with a price. For the idea of artificial companionship to become our new normal, we have to change ourselves, and in the process we are remaking human values and human connections."

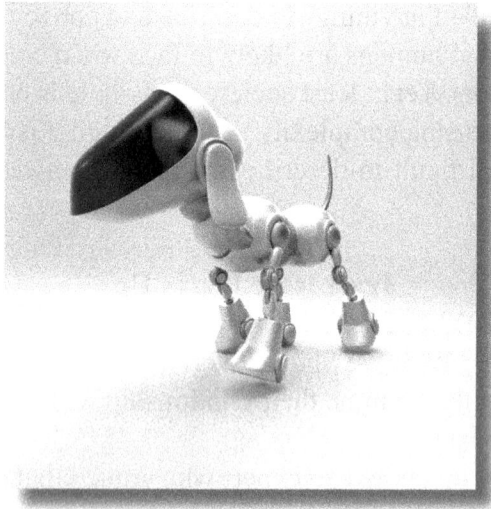

Chapter 22
Huge Issue: Robot Programming

The computer and electronic programming systems from the early days of NASA have evolved into a complex and highly specialized process.

Gone are the days when the most significant programming tasks involved the final countdown to launch--famously "10, 9, 8," and so on.

At its most basic level "programming" involves setting the criteria and mathmetical paramaters of a computer or a robot.

The programming process involves feeding pre-set information into a computer, while also commanding when and how the device will use that information.

This is a critical and urgent process, which when working properly in an "all-systems-are-go" mode will generate the desired results or performance by the device.

Critical Issues Emerge

While the programming process might seem basic and easy for people specialized in this task, such systems are likely to become highly controversial.

This aspect of the overall robotics process is so critical that when envisioning, designing and building the machines people will need to make critical decisions. Among just a handful of the many issues that electrical engineers will face:

Life and death: Particularly in instances involving a "RoboDoc," under what specific criteria will a medical robot be programming to allow the human patient to die? For instance, will robots be designed to "work less" to save low-income people, while doing more to save the wealthy? Or, just as disturbing, will patients who pay more get additional life-saving efforts than those who pay less and never receive? Perhaps just as disturbing, will these machines do less to save the lives of people in their 80s and beyond? With the world's population already swollen well past

7 billion souls, will robots be designed to take fewer measures to save the lives of extremely ill or very old individuals? Questions such as these will have to be "answered" beforehand by the people who program medical robots. Many humans likely will view this aspect of robotic programming as a cold, heartless and an even cruel process. At the early onset in the steady advancement of robotics, people need to worry that government bureaucrats could literally put your life in their hands. As briefly mentioned earlier, the Obamacare health insurance mandate has been a travesty--even well before robots begin playing an increasingly a significant role in healthcare. A government-mandated committee of appointed bureaucrats with no medical experience already is making crucial medical decisions. This cumbersome and ill-conceived process is designed to lower the government-authorized costs of specific medical procedures. Chances seem strong that critics eventually will complain that when setting the programming criteria for medical robots, officials lacking any medical knowledge whatsoever will insist that the machines do less to help seniors and the critically ill.

Treatment methods: Another critical issue likely will involve the type of medicine that healthcare robots will be programmed to practice. For instance, through the insistance of politicians and the federal government, all medical robots might be programmed to practice only mainstream, allopathic medicine. These involve dangerous and expensive BigPharma drugs. This branch of medical care involves standard treatment methods developed primarily in the Western world, systems that many people worldwide consider unnatural and in some instances far more dangerous than necessary. Under such a system, the mainstream medical industry's robots likely would use deadly, addictive and often ineffective pharmaceuticals-- while ignoring any safe, less expensive and non-addictive natural remedies that have been proven just as effective or much better. Yes, at this juncture in the advancements of medical robots, electrical engineers might seize the opportunity to ban any and all natural remedies that are administered by Homeopaths and other alternative medical professionals who avoid BigPharma products. Even now, well before the widespread rollout of advanced-level medical robots, federal agencies and university medical schools have the aforementioned propensity to favor BigPharma. Any effort to completely block natural medicine from medical robotics would involve a widespread conspiracy.

School instruction: Far more than just the medical industry, the programming of "robot teachers" might become even more controversial. Yes, officials very likely will have to face the issue of what and how robots will be programmed to teach children and adults. At this early juncture, it is far too early to forecast how many human teachers will be replaced by machines. Well into the 2010s, robot instructors already were being used on a steadily growing basis at pre-schools, elementary schools, high schools and even universities. Shockingly, however, the general public seems to have given little thought to how these instructional robots should be programmed. This specific issue could very well evolve into perhaps one of the most hotly contested challenges facing humanity during the next century. Indeed, think of a society where all robot teachers are programmed to teach the benefits of socialism, fascism, liberalism, conservatism or capitalism. Just as disturbing emerges the essential moral and religious issues. Will robots be programmed to teach or show a preference to any specific religion--or perhaps to reject all forms of religion.

Morals and values: With equal importance, what morals and value systems will robots be programmed to have--ranging from machines that "work" in the medical industry to "everyday, common and typical" robots that people own at home? Needless to say, electrical engineers or the "human bosses" who tell them what to do must program robots to display certain morals and values. In some cultures today it's considered OK or even encouraged to kill or harm people who have certain religious beliefs, or to harm individuals who are wealthy or destitute. Once again we have instances where people who program robots will need to make life-and-death decisions, essentially telling the robots how to behave in specific circumstances.

Military robots: Later on in a subsequent chapter, you'll learn much more about the advancements in destructive, deadly and extremely powerful military robots. For now, keep in mind that many people fear that "Robot Soldiers" of the near future will be able to capture, enslave or kill people in entire cities or countries within a short period. The programming of these much-feared devices might hinge on such basics as killing all male humans above age 16 or obliterating all people who have certain political, economic or ideological beliefs. Once again, the issue of military robotics generates another challenge, the need to manage the behavior of machines designed to cause widespread death and destruction.

The news media: With robots already entering journalism at a steady pace, what political ideologies will these devices be programmed to have--liberal, centrist or conservative? All this comes down to the disturbing fact that throughout history, the vast majority of people within specific societies have essentially believed "whatever they have been taught." Under this line of thinking, at least in a philosophical sense, the masses of human beings essentially are like dogs or chimpanzees--taught how to behave from their infancy and beyond. Such worries are understandable. Toddlers today already are being given cell phones, laptops, and iPads as quasi-babysitters. Think of the political indoctrination that these children will have forced-fed into their impressionable minds, particularly if robots that they play with have been programmed to spout or teach over-the-top political dogma.

Creativity and freedom: As you'll learn in much more detail in subsequent chapters, scientists are developing robots that perform highly creative tasks--which until now have been done only by humans. Within the field of robotics these "skills" will include everything from writing novels and screenplays, to painting pictures, singing and even acting in films. Quite disturbingly, if all goes as electrical engineers plan, these machines will have the capability of performing creative tasks just as well as--or likely superior to--"mere human beings." Yet will scientists program robots to take over and dominate all these creative pursuits, that until now have individually and collectively served as key hallmarks of humanity? On a similar proverbial playing field, can or will creative robots essentially rob all people of their personal freedoms? Questions like these seem logical and even necessary. After all, imagine having lifelong dreams of becoming an actor, singer or skilled writer--only to realize that robots have, can and will do far better at such pursuits than you could possibly imagine.

Financial management: As strange and other-worldly as this might seem, it's true--by early 2015 robots were already getting into the financial management industry. Amazingly, many people already were embracing such systems, allowing "automated, computer-based systems" to manage their personal portfolios. This transition began during the first decade of this century, when early-version programs such as Betterment.com developed automated systems for managing entire financial portfolios. Then, after numerous finance industry companies began similar efforts, in early 2015 the Charles Schwab wealth management service launched "Schwab Intelligent Portfolios(tm)." As of 2015, this no-fee service created diversified portfolios for people with as little as $5,000 to invest. According to the Website, "to build and manage your portfolio, Schwab Intelligent Portfolios uses an advanced algorhythm and the professional insight of the Charles Schwab Investment Advisory Inc. Team. Portfolios include up to 20 asset classes across stocks, fixed income, real estate and commodities, as well as an FDIC-insured cash component, so they're truly diversified." Remarkably, automated systems such as this have done remarkably well at diversifying accounts--while historically and consistently outperforming the financial results generated by human financial advisors. Financial companies and investment firms always use catch-all phrases such as "past performance is no indiciation of future results." Even so, in coming years, if some finance analyst forecasts are correct, human financial advisors could get phased out of the process. The key factor is that the automated robotic-style investment systems charge little or no fees. This could emerge as a "deciding factor" for major investors, particularly among those having portfolios above $10 million. Unlike most of the new automated programs, which charge little or no fees as previously stated, human financial advisors typically charge a flat annual fee of around 1 percent of the client's total portfolio. For a person with $10 million in an account, this would be about $100,000 in yearly fees. Over a 10-year period, that would add up to a whopping $1 million in total fees, assuming that the financial advisor is able to generate an annual return of at least 1 percent--necessary to maintain a minimum $10 million portfolio. So, when dealing with human financial advisors, this hypothetical investor would would need a return of at least $100,000 yearly "just to break even;" by contrast, such earnings that are "necessary just to break even" would not be required when using no-fee, automated financial advisors. Similar to the case with other forms of robotics, experts have to program the auto-investment systems. These tasks bring up a maze of additional issues, such as whether automating the entire investment process would eventually cause a catastrophic "ripple effect"--potentially obliterating world or national economies.

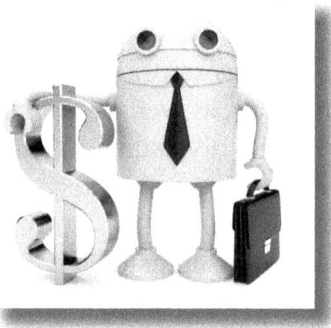

Chapter 23
Essential Robot Software

Electrical engineers and robotics experts use a process called "coded commands" to program the machines, ranging from certain mechanical devices or electronic systems.

These highly trained experts use a complex system developed to get the robots or other machines to perform certain tasks or to process data in a specified way.

The coding process involves routing or directing the data in a detailed and interwoven system. All these various criteria perform or command specialized duties, often while using specialized programming languages that depend on the type of robot. These include:

Industrial robots: These machines generally perform preset, mundane and repetitive duties in the manufacturing process. Typical tasks range from fastening screws to installing wires, or placing materials on storage platforms. Because most or all of the machine's movements are identical, the programming process is usually routine and far less complex than with other more highly specialized machines. Thus, most industrial robots generally lack any significant "decision-making" abilities, other than to follow the commands of certain routes sent to the device during the pick-up or delivery process.

Visual programming language: Usually used for somewhat more advanced robots, these programming languages sometimes start with the "desired result"--rather than the necessary data for processing commands. To do this, the engineers drag icons that designate the commands into the robot software. Then, the people rearrange the icons into a desired sequence; this is necessary to command the machine to carry out or perform tasks in the desired way.

Scripting languages: This is a highly specialized set of coding, criteria or "language" that the engineers must fully understand in order to properly program the machine to get desired results. When functioning properly, the machines process high-level programming languages "on-the-fly" or in an instant. The process is often much different from programming industrial robots, which generally are only programmed to move or perform in certain ways in almost every instance. By contrast, robots requiring highly specialized scripting languages generally require much more advanced coding and scripting languages.

Parallel languages: Somewhat more advanced robots simultaneously perform multiple tasks. These instances increase the complexity and process of software programming. To handle or regulate such increasingly complex coding tasks, electrical engineers have developed coding languages that work "in parallel" or simultaneously.

Universal programs: Although the term "universal" is rarely used in robotics programming, electrical engineers and inventors have created various command-and-control software that can be used for many types of robots. Such software or programming often serves as helpful or essential in the remote operation of machines, using hand-held devices that are controlled by people. Additionally, scientists have created point-and-click software essential in the programming of autonomous robots designed and built to operate independently from humans. Criteria for such programming also regulates the movements and tasks of mobile robots in factories.

Safety Considerations

The safety of people remains a primary concern when programming robots, even machines that perform tasks in factories. Among considerations:

Size: Many factory robots or automated machines are much larger and bulkier than people, posing a potential risk of severe injury or death to humans.

High speed: Many industrial robots work at super-fast speed, posing the possible danger of severe blunt force trauma to any person within the machines' pathways.

Pre-programming: Some robots perform only pre-programming functions, incapable of stopping or moving in a different direction when unexpectedly encountering humans.

Unexpected movements: Even if a person is mentally prepared to "run or duck" if necessary, machine movements can be far too fast for a person to escape.

For these reasons, in many instances humans are prohibited from being in the machines' "work areas." Such legitimate concerns also might emerge in non-industrial envionments, particularly instances that involve fast and sturdy machines.

Medical Environments

All of the previously mentioned programming criteria and safety considerations become critical in the creation and building of medical robots.

Builders and programmers of healthcare machines must use great care in developing efficient and safe designs. Otherwise, poorly conceived or badly programmed machines could endanger human healthcare professionals or patients.

Imagine a giant super-powerful robot arm that suddenly and unexpectedly moves toward people in rapid-fire fashion during surgery in an operating room.

This is just one of many examples of functions that can go haywire in an environment that is supposed to be sterile, calm and safe for everyone involved.

As a result, under the careful guidance of experts in medical robotics, developers of such machines must carefully create and program specialized software.

Medical Programming Advancements

Working as methodically as possible--yet at an accelerated pace--increasing numbers of medical robotics companies in recent years have been fine-tuning their programming.

Engineers have been working behind-the-scenes to improve results, although little widespread publicity has been made of these landmark developments.

According to a "Wired" magazine article published Oct. 27, 2015, at least one company was designing software to diagnose illness in humans.

If this creation by the Enlitic company works as planned, for the first time in history machines will be capable of replacing or assisting human doctors in reaching or making an accurate diagnosis.

"Enlitic won't replace radiologists," the "Wired" story said. "Instead, the software is designed to help them do their jobs more quickly and make fewer mistakes. First, it checks each file submitted to make sure the image matches what the technicians say it's supposed to be--for example, it makes sure that if an image is a left knee that it's not actually a right knee. Then, it looks for anomalies in the image."

Increasing Efficiency

From the point of reviewing the initial images, the Enlitic device provides the radiologist with a list of priorities for X-rays and routes for further examination.

If the machine performs as planned, the device will accelerate and improve the overall diagnostic process--such as detecting an aneurism for review by a cardiovascular radiologist. According to "Wired," these criteria and processes by Enlitic were just the latest example of the "deep learning" processes put into practical use by medical robots.

This marked just one example of how engineers were developing separate, independent robotic systems that use Artificial Intelligence for various medical and non-medical uses. Among the many examples:

Facebook: Started studying the use of automated, digital-based learning techniques to enable the robotics technology to develop image captions that blind people can read in brail.

Yelp: This online review and company-listing service studied the use of automated learning technology to optimize photos of restaurants and other businesses.

Skype: This online direct communication service already began using the computerized learning systems for language translation.

More Robotics Companies Emerge

Enlitic emerged as the latest in a growing number of robotics companies that sought to develop effective "learning-based" diagnostic systems for the healthcare industry.

Among the most famous was the IBM "Watson" computer, which the Memorial Sloan-Kettering Cancer Center has used for essential research.

If the progress and effectiveness of the computer-based system continued as hoped, engineers planned to transition this programming into robots.

Watson advanced to the point of giving diet and exercise advice, while other companies including "bright.md" strived to develop a computer-based learning system that specializes in helping human doctors accelerate routine appointments.

Using just as much emphasis, according to "Wired," the Enlitic process to that point served as the most significant "real-world" test of how a robotic or computer-based deep learning process enables machines to assist human doctors in diagnostics.

Advancements in Robotics Software Surge

The ongoing news about significant advancements in robotic software and robotic programming surged during the mid-2010s at never-before-seen levels.

Although the vast majority of the general public seemed to ignore or discount these stories, various news articles emphasized the fact that robotics engineers had made important discoveries for medical and non-medical uses.

When considered "as a whole," rather than merely just a single discovery, these various systems likely will impact each other. For instance, the programming advancements that enable military robots to injure more people also might motivate the developers of medical machines; these experts would develop effective gadgets for treating any wounds inflicted by the machines.

Among just some of the many hundreds of landmark discoveries or creations within robotic software and robotic programming were:

Speed writing: As reported by "Fusion" magazine, a writing software called Wordsmith(tm) enabled a journalist for the publication to post three blog listings in just three seconds. Such automated software might eventually enable doctors to use computer-based programs or robots to write detailed reports on patient visits. Several large media organizations including the Associated Press already used auto-writing software at an accelerated pace.

Cognitive intelligence: "PC Magazine" reported that the Dell computer company, has developed a "cognitive intelligence" system. According to "PC," Dell has announced that its Automated Full-Time Equivalent System is a "software agent that is programmed to perform repeatable rule-based tasks in business processes. In health care, for example, the tool can speed claims processing from 4.5 minutes down to 45 seconds, by automating many of the time-consuming and "boring tasks."

Robotic "brain cells": Scientists have developed artifical brain cells that allow robots to navigate without sensors. Amazingly, as reported by "Digital Trends" in 2015, scientists and electrical engineers created robotic software that mimics the unique ability of humans to mentally map their surroundings. People use two unique brain structures--place and grid cells-- that work en tandem to provide essential data while recalling a location. Scientists at Singapore's Agency for Science, Technology and Research (A-Star) developed a simulated version of these cells for use in robots, according to the "Technology Review" from MIT. "Using software, the team developed a simulation that mimicked the functionality of these place and grid cells," the

"Digital Trends" story said. "As their name implies, place cells recognize places in a person's environment." This natural system enables people to instinctively know their location. By mimicking this natural process, the scientists developed software that enabled a robot to navigate a 35-square meter office space using these innate-memory systems. Researchers anticipate significant advancements in robot mapping abilities as scientists continually fine-tune, improve, and expand these systems.

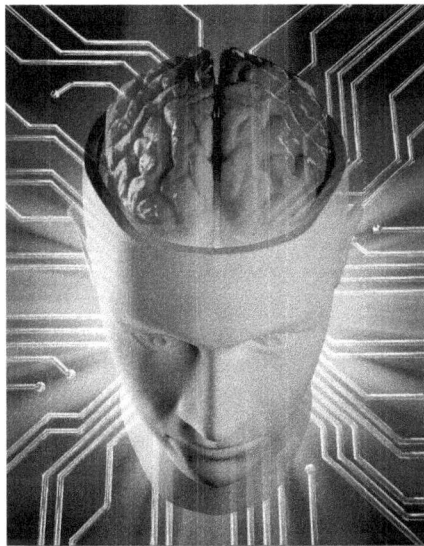

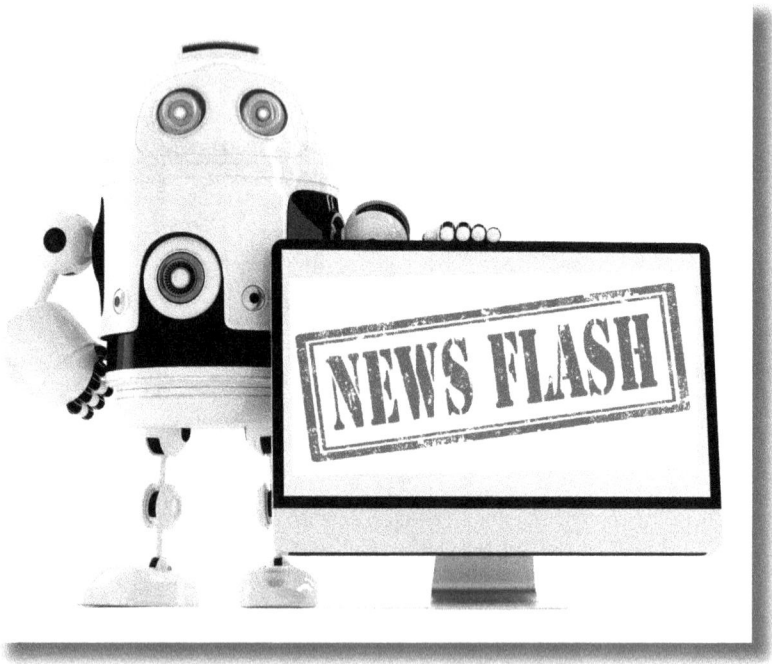

Chapter 24
News Flash:
Google Buys Robotics Companies at Rapid Pace

Amid suggestions by some people that "whoever controls the robots will rule the planet," the world's largest online company has been buying robotic companies worldwide at a steadily increasing pace in recent years.

Amazingly, the general public seems to ignore this trend. Yet without saying specifically why or how their company is purchasing lots of robotics firms, Google executives admit their effort is moving forward at a rapid pace.

Deemed among the world's largest companies by far, Google--now within a holding company called Alphabet--rapidly accelerated its diversification efforts. Every robotics company acquisition focuses on the newest technologies.

Generating several billion dollars in gross company revenue every calendar quarter, the company's executive team obviously is building for the future. The most logical and potentially profitable way to do this is by "locking in, and also owning the patents to unique and world-changing robotics technologies."

So, while the vast majority of people worldwide remained oblivious to this unstoppable trend, Alphabet continued to position itself to remain the most powerful corporation worldwide--perhaps for many generations to come.

Every Aspect of Human Life
By this point a formidable fact becomes obvious, the revelation that robotics and automated systems very soon will control or manage every aspect of human life. Everything from medical treatment to what we eat and transportation services will depend on robots. As a result, the machines might become even more essential to humanity than the Internet.

Obviously cognizant of these factors, Alphabet and its continually growing number of subsidiary companies in all likelihood will eventually dominate more than just the Web-- already done by the company's Google online division.

The "Tech Republic" technology news and analysis service listed many reasons for Google's aggressive purchase of robot companies--which involved an average of five companies yearly from 2010 to 2015. Among factors cited:

Quiet mode: After buying five robotics companies within several months, continuing a decade-long purchase trend, Alphabet remained tight-lipped about why; the company refrained from announcing its long-term intentions and strategy. Alphabet's robotics companies are highly diversified.

Differences: Besides robots with advanced Artificial Intelligence, the purchased firms include a company that developed a robot, which runs 30 miles per hour--plus other firms focused on programming such advanced machines.

Specialization: Sincre its 1998 launch, Google has been a data-driven company that heavily relies on algorithms and sensors. This is a natural carry-over into robotics, which relies on similar digital-based platforms.

Innovation: The transition into robotics is viewed by some analysts including "Tech Republic" as a natural step because Google and its parent company value innovation. This development, in turn, should continually enable Alphabet to get closer to consumers.

Significant Revenue Potential

This well-planned expansion into robotics should position Alphabet for significant revenue potential as healthcare companies and other industries become increasingly reliant on machines.

Essentially robots are like smartphones because the machines can only operate with data, special coding or Artificial Intelligence. Smartphones enable cellular companies to stay close to consumers by leveraging and capturing of data.

By latching on to robotics, Alphabet has positioned itself to benefit, particularly at the point when society fully embraces advanced or fully autonomous robotics.

"The robotics play is the same--control and influence in the last mile where data is gleaned from the physical world and activities are informed by intelligence in the cloud," Anthony Mullen, a Forrester Research senior analyst was quoted as saying in the "Tech Republic" article. "It's a good fit ... I'm not surprised it happened so quickly."

The key to Alphabet's informational success will hinge on whether society eventually accepts and embraces robotics outside of "structured environments." Those are locations such as factories where robots work in confined places.

Such a transition will depend on whether robots can or will eventually thrive and move outside of pre-designated places.

Jumping a Significant Hurdle

Numerous researchers admit that until about 2012 and beyond they had been somewhat skeptical about whether robots could move from pre-designated spaces.

But significant advancements in Artificial Intelligence began decreasing the levels of such skepticism, at least judging by dozens of news articles and reports on the subject.

Benefitting from such technological advancements, Alphabet and its Google division intensifies their robot-company buying spree.

In a sense Alphabet essentially began acquiring the bulk of available "land or space" within the realm of robotics. As a result, the company is positioned to lure human talent while seizing upon the latest unique information-storage methods.

In doing so, Alphabet has essentially been playing a proverbial chess game with the entire world. Along the way, these companies position themselves to emerge as winners when the expected transitions click into full gear.

Society Might Benefit

A steadily increasing number of business and robotics industry analysts seem to believe the Alphabet effort could eventually generate long-term benefits for society.

This is particularly true involving crisis response robots purchased and under development by various Alphabet robotics companies. These included machines developed to respond to the 2011 nuclear disaster in Fukushima, Japan.

Much more far-reaching has been Alphabet's significant leadership role in envisioning, developing and building driverless cars.

While numerous automobile companies including Tesla aggressively strive to play "catch-up" with their own driverless automobile efforts, Alphabet likely will continue to play a leadership role in this admirable quest.

The prize for the primary "winners" likely will be huge profits thanks to a long-term lock on technologies; transportation services and consumers increasingly rely on such advancements.

How Data is Used

Unlike standard software which remains inert or at a fixed location, standard robotics transform information into movement or action.

The "information age" that began to emerge and progress through the last half of the 20th Century is likely to change, transform and blossom as a result.

Rather than merely humans collecting vital and nessary data, by amassing and processing information themselves, robots should be able to do this faster and with greater efficiency.

Very soon, gone will be the days when people had to brave dangerously extreme cold to dig into arctic ice to collect samples, or to venture near active volcanoes for conducting scientific research. In fact, some of these achievements are already happening.

Even more promising, if all goes as planned, very soon the

analysis of newly collected data will be almost instant. Over time this should enable people or robots to respond faster to essential, dangerous or extremely critical situations.

Boston Dynamics Acquisiton
Perhaps Alphabet's most controversial robot company purchase involved Boston Dynamics, producer of military machines hailed by some people as "spectacular and terrifying." According to a 2013 article in "The Verge," the wonky looking Boston Dynamics robots with funny gates have "mind-blowing capabilities."

Various news reports said that the purchase at an undisclosed price included the robot company's pre-existing contract with the previously mentioned U.S. Defense Advanced Research Projects Agency (DARPA).

Boston Dynamics rapidly began specializing in military robotics in 1992, after the company was spun off from the Massachusetts Institute of Technology.

One of its most famous robots, aptly named BigDog, works efficiently in moving ice and snow. Other Boston Dynamics projects remain somewhat secretive, other than robots like PETMAN, described by "The Verge" as an "eerily convincing humanoid," and Cheetah, an animal-like robot that runs fast--up to 29 miles per hour at last report.

Tech Experts Appluad Alphabet's Move
Although Alphabet's transition into robotics initially generated a battery of jokes on Skynet, according to "Popular Science" magazine, this burgeoning industry's experts gave a surprisingly positive reaction.

"Of course, it's part of our business to tell everyone how great we think robotics is," Matt Mason, director of Carnagie Mellon's Robotics Institute was quoted as saying in the "Popular Science" article. "But this is the kind of commitment that transcends any sort of BS or rhetoric."

Even more promising from a business perspective, Alphabet's move into robotics has been viewed as a strong signal to start-up companies that the time has definitely arrived to start or grow such ventures.

On the downside, however, some observers admit they worry that by controlling a growing number of robotic companies, Alphabet is well positioned to dominate and amass the best human minds in the industry.

Another primary fear here is that these researchers will develop and create significant robotic advancements in secret.

Streams of Alphabet Robot Companies

Amid Alphabet's non-stop robot company buying spree averaging from five to 10 businesses since 2010, the firm's has many unique ventures. Among them:

Bot & Dolly: Specializing in motion control, plus filming the affects of gravity, this firm creates an illusion of weightlessness by using four separate cameras. Although some people might view this firm's film industry experience as a negative, the company's technology might help improve existing industrial robots.

Meka Robotics: Known primarily for its "M1 Mobile Manipulator," this system specializes in unique Series Elastic Actuators--unique and necessary spring devices between robotic joints and motors. Over time, such systems likely will emerge as vital for generating realistic head movements in humanoid machines. The firm's specialty focuses on arms and manipulators, characteristics designed to ensure safe environments for people.

Boston Dynamics: Briefly mentioned earlier, this firm specializes in military robots that feature super-powerful leg movements and strength. Autonomous robots that never require human interaction in the future will need these attributes in a highly effective and reliable manner--particularly for machines with "legs."

Holomni: Still striving to create momentous and useful features, this company specializes partly on developing "omnidirectional wheels" that enable machines to move in multiple directions. Some analysts believe this venture enables Alphabet to diversify in instances where such mobility proves more effective than human-like lower limbs.

SCHAFT Inc.: Known primarily for its "S-One" brand robot, SCHAFT is also credited with developing liquid-cooled electric actuators. This Tokyo-based company's products might generate huge demand after winning first place in U.S. government DARPA robotics challenge trials. "Popular Science" has said that SCHAFT's monster actuators seem to compliment or overlap with "Boston Dynamics' beefy actuators." This leads some robotics industry analysts to believe that Alphabet is trying to have a key role in the development and eventual use of every kind of robotic technology.

Redwood Robotics: Within three years of its 2012 launch, this firm remained busy focusing on efforts to create, build and supply manufacturers with reliable robot arms. Several firms combined to join this venture, including Willow Garage, SRI International, and Meka Robotics. Some robotic industry observers believe that the firms will pool their resources of existing technologies that collectively generate extremely safe robots that require little energy.

Industrial Perception Inc.: This firm specializes in creating and building robots that quickly and effectively sort through stacks of materials such as boxes. Assuming that technological advances continued as expected, over time the company would use stereo cameras, enabling robots to find, retrieve and move specific materials. Right away this might boost the effectiveness of industrial robots, while also improving the capabilities needed by almost every class of moving AI machines. These would range form airborne drones and first-responder robots being funded by the Pentagon.

Autofuss: Working with its previously mentioned sister company, Bot & Dolly, this firm specializes in creating highly complex, visually compelling advertisements. This video production company has received relatively little publicity, leading to an unverified theory that perhaps Alphabet will make the venture an essential part of its broad robotics business and marketing plan.

Industry Consolidation

Far too numerous to list here in full, Alphabet's numerous robotic companies represent an industry consolition.

At least in a broad sense, this effort is somewhat similar to the rapid spread and advancement of the automobile industry in the early 1900s.

Back then particulalry in the Detroit area, dozens of fledging car companies sprouted; this happened thanks to entrepreneurs who raced to build the best, most effective and affordable transportation technologies.

A handful of the earliest automobile manufacturers strived to create the best, most profitable and in-demand technologies; the Ford Motor Company emerged as the most successful. That firm's founder, Henry Ford, excelled in adopting new innovations--particularly the assembly line. This revolutionary manufacturing system enabled groups of factory workers to specialize in specific chores; these tasks were done as newly formed automobiles moved on conveyor belts past the employees' work stations.

By comparison, as of late 2015 Alphabet had still not announced how--if at all--the company might try to merge and centralize the robotics creation and manufacturing industry. Yet with the brightest robotics experts and the best new technologies, consolidation into a specialized robot manufacturing facility seemed to emerge as the company's most logical and profitable next step.

Competition Breeds Success

Amid this broad international transition, streams of non-Alphabet robotics companies continued to emerge.

Scientists, engineers and other exeprts work together and

individually to advance robotics; these people are employed by companies, universities and governments worldwide.

At least in some ways, this surge toward "a proverbial treasure" resembled the great and famous California Gold Rush of 1849. Back then, people from around the world streamed to the Golden State in hopes of generating quick riches.

Yet within the first several years the "easiest pickings" had already been pulled from that future state's streams and rivers. This left the vast majority of these new Californians penniless; only a handful of them attained financial wealth. Many companies reaping the biggest rewards were firms that supplied these people with necessities that ranged from mining material to food and clothing.

By comparison, those making the biggest profit from the rapidly emerging robotics trend of today likely will be:

Suppliers: Companies that supply the robot manufacturers with the necessary materials, ranging from unique metals and wiring, to plastics and robot-building facilities.

Investors: Individuals or firms that invest early in robotics developers and manufacturers that eventually become highly profitable or dominate the industry.

Experts: As briefly mentioned earlier, the people most likely to get the best jobs will be those who earn undergraduate or advanced degrees in: metallurgy; electrical engineering; mathematics; physics; and other robotics specialties.

Entrepreneurs: Working behind the scenes and initially with little or no publicity, entrepreneurs might envision, create and actually develop specialized materials or systems that eventually become necessary to the entire robotics industry. The key examples here might be the early successful innovators in Internet-related industries. From the 1980s to the early 2000s, these included firms that initially started in garages of small residential homes or at small offices. Besides Alphabet's predecessor, Google, the most famous of these include Apple Computer co-founded by the late Stephen Jobs; Microsoft, founded by Bill Gates; and

Facebook, founded by Mark Zuckerberg. Each of these people became billionaires thanks to their willingness to take risks, coupled with their firms' technological developments deemed necessary by society.

By comparison, the development of robotics is now at the equivalent of where the Internet was in the late 1980s and early 1990s; Internet-related innovators back then solidified and patented the bulk of their new technologies before the Web surged in international popularity from the mid-1990s and beyond.

Similarly, the robotics industry is now positioned to boom in a similar way, at least judging by many of the aforementioned news stories and scientific reports. During the next few decades, if advancements continue as planned, many people are likely to tell themselves: "I wish I had bought a certain robotic company stock back in the 2010s," or "I could have been the person who developed a much-needed robotic software in my garage way back then--why didn't I?" While keeping these various interlinking factors into perspective, it is quite possible to assume that at this very moment budding entrepreneurs are working in garages or cheap make-shift facilities to create and build milestone robotics systems.

Patent Filing Accelerates

The necessary patents to lock in the rights to these vital and necessary robotic technologies is likely to surge at an ever-increasing pace through the 2020s.

Every step of the way, society's race toward robotics is likely to generate complex legal challenges--somewhat similar to those that hampered start-up Internet-related firms.

Indeed, the race to start the Web industry sparked intense litigations, some stretching on for more than a decade among warring companies that battled for domination.

Seemingly every major firm within that sector that eventually achieved multi-billion dollar annual revenues got ensnared in such legal disputes. These ranged from Apple and

Microsoft to Facebook and many more.

Although the age-old saying remains true, that "the business of business is--business," in today's increasingly hostile and litigious environment the process invariably involves "legal war."

Legal Battles Will Erupt

If the past serves as an indiction, intense and highly publicized legal litigation will erupt among robotics companies in the 2020s.

With equal intensity, consumers will likely enter these confrontations as well--with average people alleging that they have been financially or physically harmed by product defects.

In all of these instances the prizes will either become a court-mandated authorization to dominate the robotics indusry, or financial windfalls--or both.

These burgeoning factors in turn in all likelihood will spawn a new legal battleground for lawyers. Many of today's attorneys specialize in everything from libel law to divorce litigation and personal injury.

Add robotics issues to this, and lawyers as an overall sector likely will find themselves positioned for huge potential financial windfalls--at least until the point when robots eventually replace human attorneys.

Such a paradoxical outcome might seem like an odd mix of humor and serious groundbreaking case law. In a rather quirky yet possible scenario, envision a system where robots serving as lawyers in courtrooms defend--or even litigate against--the same companies that produced them. Such bizarre scenarios might occur much faster than many people can envision.

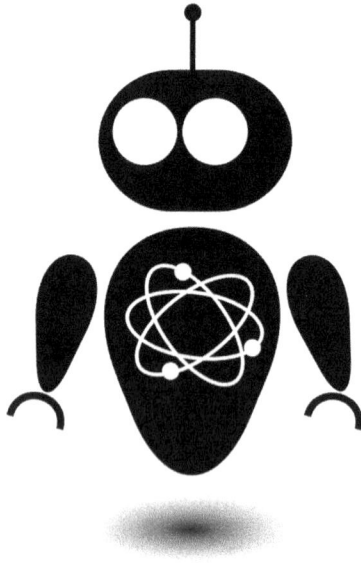

Chapter 25
Extreme Fear of Robots

Hospitals, medical clinics and businesses worldwide have failed to recognize the fact that millions of people worldwide have an extreme fear of robots.

Such fears emerge as a natural and instinctive part of the human psyche, a condition that psychologists call "automatonophobia."

This involves far more than merely robots, but also any type of "sentient being"--manmade objects that seem to have human characteristics.

These typically range from ventriloquist dummies, puppets and dolls to scarecrows, mannequins and wax creatures.

For many hundreds or thousands of years, people suffering from "automatonophobia" have suffered from extreme panic attacks.

Hospitals and Medical Clinics Failed

Hospital administrators and scientists tragically have overlooked this condition when pursuing plans to introduce robots into health care facilities.

The percentage of people from this adverse condition seems unknown, reportedly perhaps about only 1 percent of the world population.

The adverse impact on society could be extreme, particularly in medical environments where some patients already become overly stressed.

Even with just 1 percent of people suffering from automatonophobia, the robots might endanger the mental health of patients who already have enough problems.

This adverse psychological condition has become so pervasive that in recent years some scientists and psychologists have started calling the specific fear of machines "robophobia."

Much More Study Needed

Far more research is needed on this little-known issue, which still had failed to catch the attention of the mainstream media in the mid-2010s. Among the possible symptoms that reportedly still need to be verified were:

Heart attacks: The sudden or unexpected appearance of a robot might cause extreme panic, leading to a potentially fatal or life-changing heart attack.

Blood pressure: The possibility of sudden increases in blood pressure might create circulation problems, heart ailments or even potentially fatal strokes.

Asthma: Whether "real" or unwarranted, excessive fear sometimes leads to extreme or potentially catastrophic breathing difficulties, including asthma.

Mental function: All sense of logic theoretically disappears when the person's thought processes get "locked in fear."

Avoid Rush to Judgment

Any assertation of the aforementioned symptoms remains speculative because much more research is needed on this subject.

Electrical engineers and administrators of health care facilities need to take pro-active measures early--before robots permeate the medical industry.

All along, some officials familiar with this condition in recent years have quickly labeled any fear of robots as "extreme, unnecessary and illogical."

These experts insist that consumers and everyday citizens have absolutely nothing to fear from these machines, carefully programmed to help rather than hurt people.

Yet merely saying such things as "you need to act rational" likely would do little or nothing to help people suffering from automatonophobia involving robots. The difficulty in devising adequate treatments and preventions stem from the fact that most people suffering from this condition lose their short- or long-term ability to think rationally.

Avoid Blaming the Media

Some observers have gone so far as to blame the entertainment industry and the news media for spreading misinformation about the apparent dangers of robots.

Movies, television shows, and even news stories during the past century have exacerbated or created irrational and unnecessary fears.

Many such tales have been characterized by fantasy accounts of a robotic apocalypse or the enslavement of and extinction of humanity--the violence and kidnappings instigated by such machines.

The joint announcement by internationally famous physicist Stephen Hawkings and other luminaries might have only served to intensify such worries on a broad scale.

As a result, many people--particularly teens and young adults who grew up with such intense stories--might view robots as "our future overlords, rather than our helpers."

Medical Industry Suffers

As robots permeate society, almost every type of industry is likely to suffer from such fears--whether warranted or unjustified.

The most severe and problematic instances are likely to impact the healthcare industry, perhaps far more than other business sectors. Among potential challenges:

Sudden bursts: A need to control people who suddenly flail their limbs in seemingly every direction, screaming nonsense while displaying irrational behavior.

Surgeries: Sudden physical fights with human medical personnel, starting when the patient realizes that the "surgeon" is actually a robot.

Irrational thoughts: Somewhat mirroring paranoid schizophrenia, unfounded worries might emerge--such as a possibility that the "RoboDoc" will surreptitiously implant dangerous objects into the patient's body.

Confusion: The patient might fear that any or all of the hospital's human personnel are actually devilish robots, when in fact none of--or only a handful--of the medical "workers" are machines.

Relatives: Such sudden, disruptive and dangerous outbursts might also involve human relatives visiting patients treated at hospitals or clinics.

Visiting this "Uncanny Valley"

Perplexed and somewhat dismayed themselves by such reactions, some scientists and sociologists have started referring to this dilemma as an "uncanny valley."

This designates a type of serious condition that is extremely difficult to pinpoint and define, conditions where the root mental triggers are difficiult to identify and treat.

An "Inverse" magazine science and technology article in October 2015 recognized and chronicled the many subtleties of this difficult-to-define condition.

"Basically as a robot more looks and acts like a human being, we increasingly empathize and relate to it--until a certain point is crossed, where suddenly the robot takes on an eerie quality that is too human," the article said.

While the specific reasons for this might remain unclear, the article said, "it might be an extraordinary knee-jerk reaction where our autonomous senses--specifically, the ones scanning and evaluating potential mates--detects features in someone (or in this case *something*) that raises flags and points to a bad mate.

"It might also be an instinctual response to seeing something that goes against conventional norms, or our heads trying to resolve the cognitive dissonance that comes with conflicting perceptual cues (i.e. something that looks and sounds human, but which you know isn't really human.)"

"Welcome, Doctor Frankenstein"

These various factors converge in a dilemma that the

widely acclaimed late author Isaac Asimov once labeled as the "Frankenstein Complex." This involves a fear that something made by people ultimately will attack its creator.

This aptly named scenario is reminiscent of Mary Shelley's famed novel where a monster comprised of dead body parts murders its creator, Doctor Frankenstein.

Such scenarios tap deep into the essence of basic fears, especially worries that humans would build a powerful object that humanity fails to fully understand.

These concerns hinge on worries that humans are irresponsible or even reckless if attempting to build something as mysterious and dangerous as a high-functioning robot.

Compounding these challenges multi-fold comes the additional notion that robots are just as infallible and imperfect as humans--prone to make life-altering or even fatal mistakes. Strangely, when viewed or perceived by a fairly intelligent human, "the irrational somehow seems to become rational--in a world where absolutely nothing seems to make any logical sense as a result."

Blame the Entertainment Industry

On a broad scale such worries have been spread and infused into the human psyche by numerous popular movies featuring indestructible robots.

The most popular and notorious of these films range from the "Terminator" films to the "Matrix" trilogy, all featuring powerful, deadly robots that turn against humans.

Each of these instances and dozens more, from popular books to TV shows, feature storylines where people struggle to save humanity from extinction.

Taking an opposite but equally disturbing approach was the British-American science fiction TV series, "Humans," which premiered in June 2015. The show dealt with the emotional impacts of the blurred lines between humans and robots.

Some disturbing yet magnetic subplots in "Humans"

involved robots that were extremely terrified of people. The machines are programmed to have emotions, but these devices must face the realization that heartless humans eventually will destroy them.

The Real-World Medical Environment

All of these various factors and scenarios lead to a disturbing revelation, the difficult-to-ignore fact that human doctors and medical professionals very likely will face extreme challenges due to automatonophobia and robophobia.

Obviously, human doctors, nurses and other highly trained health care experts already have enough important responsibilities--rather than needing to face the additional challenge of patients going into sudden panic attacks. The added need to control irrational fears sparked by robophobia only compounds an already-difficult challenge.

Rather that essentially waiting until it is "too late," past the point where tragedies occur in hospitals and medical clinics, authorities need to be pro-active now--early on in the overall process of bringing robots into healthcare environments. Among the many suggested preventative measures:

Training: Particularly while attending medical school or nursing school, or during residencies, medical professionals need to learn immediate response methods to sudden outbursts or shock--suffered by patients with robophobia.

Peaceful Environments: Use soothing music, appropriate pharmaceuticals and creative interior building designs to help put patients in a relaxed, soothing mood.

Coordination: Adopt a unified or universal system where doctors, engineers and medical facility operators work together in the development of robots and environments designed to instill a sense of safety.

Introduction: Gradually introduce the robots to patients, thereby enabling the people to gradually become accustomed to the machines. Such sensible steps should be made on a well-planned basis, rather than quickly putting robots into patient areas immediately before scheduled medical procedures such as surgery.

Programming: Program or direct the software that operates advanced robots to accommodate for and adapt to the possibility that a patient might suffer from irrational fear.

Specific Causes Unknown

Even with today's modern medicine, the specific causes of automatonophobia and robophobia remain unknown, at least according to a variety of sources.

Until authorities pinpoint the specific triggers of this condition, the Rise of the Robots likely will cause major challenges thorughout society.

Thus, people everywhere are unwittingly entering what some people call a "slippery slope," a dangerous point of no return. Such problems very likely generate a continual catch-up effort to control the problem.

"People often become terrified of anything that they fail to understand," I sometimes tell patients. "So, the biggest way to jump this proverbial hurdle is to launch an eduction system, essentially telling the world that 'robots are here to help.'"

On the flip side of this issue, however, emerges a potential propaganda system that could fool people--denying them the truth that some robots are "made to kill."

"The Naked Ape"

This steadily increasing dilemma brings to mind the hit 1967 book "The Naked Ape," which chronicled the fact that human beings are actually "mere animals"--although technology has far surpassed a single person's ability to cope with the world.

Even way back then the author, zoologist and ethologist Desmond Morris recognized the dangers that modern technology imposes on people.

Although humans are vastly more intelligent than other animals, in a biological sense, we "mere people" have the same basic instinctive urges as such "lower-level" creatures. Like other animals, our natural desires include food, companionship with our own kind, and a internal yearning for basic comforts such as shelter.

Morris argued that human beings took a long time to evolve, perhaps thousands or even millions of years. Yet the sudden advent of robots brings a perceived danger; mankind supposedly would need many years to adapt psychologically to new advanced technologies.

Such theories represented forward-thinking by Morris, who proclaimed his philosophy at a time when the most famous new technologies included nuclear bombs, TV, the advent of early computers and the then-burgeoning space program.

Challenges Increased Multi-Fold

The extreme challenges that technology poses to mankind have surged many times over since the release of "The Naked Ape."

Like this or not, vastly improved communications systems, the Internet and eventually robots will continually force all people to quickly adapt--particularly human doctors.

This could prove formidable, largely because from the perspective of many physicians, using mere machines to handle health care strikes the psyche as mysteriously unnatural.

Of course, at this point no in-depth studies seem available on this theory. Even so, the very notion of putting our lives in the hands of machines has become somewhat ludicrous.

After all, because we arrive naked into this world, the very notion that we should be cared for and fully rely upon machines for our very survival somehow seems unfathomable and ridiculous.

Warning: There is "No Turning Back"

For more than a century, many people have proclaimed that "if God had meant man to fly, people would have been born with wings." Such statements invariably come to mind when commercial airliners crash or sustain severe mechanical problems.

Yet as almost everyone seems to know, these days there essentially is "no turning back," because society has reached a point where humans depend on airplanes.

Similarly, very soon there will be almost no way to remove robotic devices and AI digital software systems from the healthcare industry and other essential business sectors.

Our fears will fail to do us any good, in an unavoidable and unstoppable situation. Like it or not, in this regard the healthcare business is essentially about to face challenges similar to those facing commercial airlines.

Despite fears of flying that they might have, any person today who wants or needs to travel overseas fast must overcome or block such personal worries. Very soon similar challenges are likely to engulf the entire healthcare industry, at least where fear is concerned.

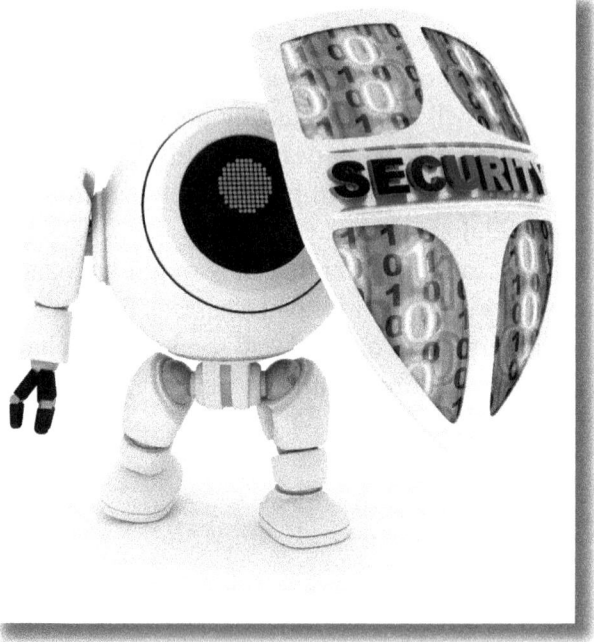

Chapter 26
Another Extreme Danger: Criminals Hacking Robots

One of the biggest challenges facing the medical indusry and all other major business sectors during the next century involves "the hacking of robots."

These days domestic and international computer and Internet hacking incidents generate headlines worldwide.

According to news reports, every major U.S. government agency has been targeted of hackers, some in clandestine operations run by other countries. Major industries and large corporations have been similarly victimized.

Invariably in many of these instances the Web security experts have blamed the fact that the "Internet essentially was built and created the wrong way to begin with." Experts contend that when gradually building the infrastructure for the Internet from the 1960s through the 1980s, scientists failed to realize how huge of a role that the Web eventually would play in everyone's life.

As a result the Internet's core infrastructure has many vulnerabilities that hackers use to their advantage. The problem has become so pervasive that experts say that virtually every Website, email system and computer infrastructure is "hackable and highly vulernable."

Worsening this horrendous problem many times over, scientists worldwide are racing at lightning speed to create highly advanced robots and Artificial Intelligence. Concerns seem to be increasing that perhaps these new technologies are charging ahead far too fast, failing to build adequate and reliable "anti-hacking systems for robots."

Hackers Might Endanger Health
The entire healthcare industry could soon be compromised,

unless reliable measures are invented and implemented to prevent the hacking of machines.

Such a tragic outcome could endanger the lives and the health of all patients.

Worsening matters, the vast majority of the aforementioned medical robots and automated healthcare systems could become vulnerable to such attacks.

To help put this into clear perspective, envison today's modern air transportation systems. Every time people go into airports to travel by commercial airliners, these individuals are required to go through X-ray machines and have thier baggage searched, even if they dislike or detest these procedures.

Mandatory airport security systems worldwide have become major hassles for travelers. Government-mandated safety and security protocols requires all passengers to arrive at airports several hours earlier than their flights' scheduled departures.

Then, adding to these hassles multi-fold, the passengers are forced to stand in long lines--sometimes for lengthy periods stretching for well over one hour.

By comparsion, the healthcare industry likely could very soon face similar restrictions, particularly if electrical engineers rush too fast in developing and designing medical robots--without creating and installing effective anti-hacking procedures.

Disturbing Security Requirements Emerge

Getting checked into hospitals or just visiting those facilities is already mentally taxing on many people, well before the widespread surge of robotics into those institutions.

The very essence of the words "hospital" or "clinic" are supposed to designate peaceful and safe places, where highly trained medical personnel strive to help make visitors and patients feel as tranquil as possible. The perceived attributes of peace and safety are so essential to the healthcare industry that some of these facilities hire architects and interior designers who specialize in creating calm, soothing environments.

Such efforts could get pushed aside at an increasingly disturbing pace, assuming that robots eventually enter the industry full-force as planned. The situation would be exacerbated multi-fold if robot hacking surges. Among the many possible outcomes:

Long lines: Patients with non-emergency conditions and visitors would have to endure long lines to enter the facilities, similar to the famously cumbersome process that travelers must endure at airports.

Security checks: Under worst-case scenarios, all visitors--including doctors and healthcare personnel--would have to go through X-ray devices when entering these buildings.

Bag checks: All bags including purses and containers would be subject to security checks; security guards would search through personal items.

Computer monitoring: Every person entering would have to provide an authorized government identification badge. Guards would imput this data into an Internet-based system, monitoring and recording the "coming and going" of each person.

Monitoring devices: A worst-case scenario would involve electronic, computerized and Web-based monitoring devices--placed on all visitors and even the facilities' personnel. Such a system would continually monitor each person's movements throughout the medical facility, including visitor restrooms and patient rooms.

When Fears Become "Justified"

The aforementioned possible security procedures are purely speculative. Yet such mandatory regulations are likely to be considered if overall security involving medical robots becomes uncontrollable.

Instances of automatonophobia or robotophobia might seem fully justified in such situations, as people encounter legitimate reasons for fear.

Although President Franklin Delano Roosevelt famously said, "We have nothing to fear but fear itself," most reasonable people could never be blamed for feeling terrorized in such situations--not just by hackers or robots, but also by "Big Brother."

Some politicians have argued in recent years that people must give up certain freedoms, so that the government can protect all law-abiding citizens.

Meantime, another disturbing question emerges, namely, "Does the government truly have our best interest at heart, or is the government currupt and overstepping its bounds?"

Quite disturbingly, under such situations many people could begin distrusting government and medical corporations, just as much as they dislike hackers and robots.

Evolutionary Hacking Process

Breaking into the inner workings of robots and changing their functions involves a far different type of hacking process than the strategies that criminals typically use to disrupt or steal from Web-based applications.

When breaking into Websites or snaking into other people's computers, hackers essentially are like burglars entering private property. Once inside their targets, these criminals steal vital data or install malware that moves the damage to other devices.

By contrast, the hacking of robots often entails taking a machine and retooling or reprogramming its functions. In a sense, this is like taking a 1957 Chevrolet and putting a much different type of engine into the vehicle; this changes the car's function.

Additionally, "breaking into robots" to change their pre-programmed functions or to steal data also can entail standard Web-based methods. The specific strategy chosen by hackers will depend on whether the machine uses Internet communications.

Both Web hackers and robot hackers continually develop and test creative new ways to destroy or disrupt their targets while also stealing or manipulating data. Working in teams or alone, many hackers consider their ongoing and non-stop efforts as a full-time job.

As a result, when creating and building robots or automated systems for the healthcare industry--or for any other business sectors--engineers must remain vigilant in installing anti-hacking devices.

Disturbing Results Might Occur

The possibility of robot hacking emerges as particularly disturbing in medical environments. Hackers might jerry-rig robotic devices in efforts to kill patients, severely injure people or make the hospital or doctors a target for lawsuits.

In an "Irish Examiner" article, a university lecturer in medical sociology, Myles Balfe, said the good news is that the vast majority of robots throughout society will lack advanced function. If true, most machines would handle domestic chores such as cleaning dishes, mowing lawns or scrubbing barbecues.

Even so, Balfe is among experts who concede that through the 21st Century some robots will become a responsive part of the world's communications systems--with numerous machines featuring at least some degree of intelligence.

"They likely will be designed with limitations in mind, in terms that their behavior will be guided by by algorithms and programming built into it--which will reflect societal standards and laws," Balfe said. "However, the history of technology consistently teaches us that what people do with technology in practice is often very different from what designers intended. Users can take technologies down unexpected paths."

These factors, in turn, should motivate robotics engineers to become increasingly vigilant in implementing anti-hack systems. This is especially true, Balfe said, because "the more expensive the robot--the greater the risk of catastrophe if it is hacked."

Catastrophic Changes Made By Non-Experts

Worsening the dangers even more at heatlhcare institutions

or other businesses, inexperienced or unauthorized employees might intentially try to modify the robots.

Although well-intentioned in some instances, these personnel might unintentionally "do the wrong thing" or "flip an incorrect switch."

Long before the advent of robots, mechanics and employees assigned to "repair things" in various industries have inadvertently triggered severe accidents. The most notorious incidents have ranged from NASA's January 1986 Challenger disaster that killed seven crew members to airline crashes caused by mechanical difficulties.

Medical robots that the healthcare industry initially adopts will become outdated or begin to break due to normal wear and tear. But what if by that point the robots' original manufacturers have discontinued services, filed bankruptcy or closed?

Businesses of all types, particularly hospitals and medical clinics, need to prepare long beforehand for such scenarios. Otherwise, inexperienced or unqualified personnel could eventually try to retool or repair the machines--sometimes with disastrous results.

Society's Obsession With Hacking

The Rise of the Robots within medical environments and throughout society comes at a pivotal juncture in history when mankind has become obsessed by hacking.

During the summer of 2015 "Mr. Robot," a new USA Network show about a hacker, skyrocketed into an overnight ratings sensation. The show's sudden popularity indicated that society had already become mesmerized by hackers--almost to the point of romanticizing such crime.

Portrayed by actor Rami Malek, the show's main character, Elliot Anderson, works during the day as a cybersecurity engineer. At night he hacks into other people's lives; Anderson strives to infiltrate a coalition of hackers led by "Mr. Robot," portrayed by actor Christian Slater.

The show seemed to have increased the interest in hacking computers, the Internet and robots. Yet whether the viewers' obsession with the show would actually motivate people to increase hacking attempts remained a matter of speculation.

In a disturbing trend that seemed never-ending, since the beginning of the 21st Century some top Internet company executives have even encouraged their friends or employees to become expert hackers. Perhaps the most notorious of these incidents involved Facebook Founder Mark Zuckerberg, whose affiliation with hacking teams was chronicled in the hit 2010 Colombia Pictures film, "The Social Network."

Popularity Breeds Copy-Cats

A sad fact emerges between these two converging trends, the Rise of the Robots and the steady or increased popularity of hacking.

Even a casual observer might assume that very soon hackers will make disrupting medical robots their self-assigned, full-time job.

In all likelihood, such nefarious activities will be carried out by people who break into medical facilities, employees of those institutions, workers at robot-manufacturing businesses, and also by people skilled at breaking into Internet data systems.

The dangers could arguably intensify even more as standard Internet hackers strive to crack the United State's government database containing the personal medical information of all patients treated nationwide. Doctors, hospitals and medical clinics must input highly sensitive and personal healthcare info into a mandatory database as required by Obamacare; this must be done every time a patient visits a doctor, hospital or clinic.

Getting this sensitive information could generate a pathway for hackers to attack specific patients via "corrupted" robots, or even blackmail--a threat to pubicly disclose personal medical information unless ransoms are paid.

Hackers Target Vulnerabilities

The liberal mainstream news media that supported Obamacare made little or no mention of this. In the summer of 2015, Internet security experts issued what they called a "disturbing warning" about severe vulnerabilities in the national healthcare database.

A paradoxial and disturbing situation arises in part because bureaucrats have named the database "Midas," in honor of a famed god from Greek Mythology whose touch turned things into gold. Critics fear that weaknesses in the system's infrastructure; this vulnerability could severaly compromise the safety and personal information of millions of people.

Recklessly storing the information in cyberspace, the Obama administration required that the data include the most sensitive personal data imaginable. Besides Social Security numbers and birthdates, the information includes addresses, employment status, financial accounts and highly personal or sensitive health information.

Irresponsible bureaucrats have insisted that this ill-conceived information storage system is crucial in the smooth operations of the mandatory insurance marketplace. When initially launching Midas, officials assured the public that the data would only be used to determine a patient's eligibility--while having a limited impact on personal privacy.

However, without any public notice, authorities also began storing this sensitive information for additional reasons that never have been fully disclosed.

Incompetence Leads to Vulnerabilities

The incompetent and unprofessional way that the Obama administration stored the inforatmion led to a severe security weakness--a serious flaw that eventually will carry over into medical robotics.

You see, advanced robots that eventually enter the medical

industry will rely on the same database initially used by human doctors and medical professionals.

One of the most potentially catastrophic flaws stems from the disturbing fact that officials plan to indefiniteily store the information. This contrasts with standard longtime medical procedures that mandated such data be kept for only limited periods.

As reported in June 2015 by the "Western Journalism" publication, former Social Security Commissioner Michael Astrue complains that the government had no justification for permanently storing the information.

Worsening matters, Astrue said, the government "illegally" added information to Midas by inputting personal data collected by state-run Obamacare facilities--without first asking people for permission to do that.

Trending Toward Disaster

As previously stated, all major federal agencies have been targeted by hackers. The IRS information system even got cracked open, although that agency supposedly has the most secure data storage systems. Many of these clandestine activities occurred during 2013-14, when hackers compromised the credit card information of hundreds of millions of people.

"There have been growing concerns by watchdog groups since the inception of Midas, and its implementation without proper safeguards" the "Western Journalism" article said. "The system has shown weaknesses. With major corporations being hacked, it is no wonder people may be more than a little concerned about a singular system holding that much information."

All this started occurring amid a "perfect storm," as literally 1.5 million Websites could easily be found in standard Google searches--simply by typing in the phrase "how to hack robots." As hackers have consistently proven, any manmade system can eventually be cracked by people eager to carry out such devilish plans.

Besides the multi-trillion-dollar medical industry, other businesses sectors that could simultaneously become vulnerable due to robotics and Web-based applications include food production, transportation, and even national security systems.

At this relatively early juncture, some Websites are eagerly and openly providing computer codes specifically designed for hacking specific brands or types of robots. Once again, society has been forced to deal with technological advancements that invariably lead to a critical increase in security flaws.

Use Hackers for Good Purposes

Rather than merely concentrating on the negatives, society and especially manufacturers of medical robots should "use hackers to our advantage."

Numerous Web security experts in recent years have proclaimed that society generally has a negative view of hackers--perceiving all of them as "bad people."

To the contrary, however, some online security professionals insist that only a small percentage of people with superior hacking skills are criminals.

Among those making this claim is Michael Bazzell, technical consultant for the "Mr. Robot" TV show. Bazzell spent a decade working for the FBI's cyber crime division; he now works as a cyber crime security consultant for private industry.

Discussing the hacking issue in 2015 with "Forbes" magazine, Bazzell insisted that the mere mention of the word "hacker" has negative connotations. This occurred because an unholy perception about these people seems to have stuck in the public mindset.

Turn a "Negative" into a "Positive"

To prevent any misconceptions, Bazzell would like people to create a new word that designates or separates specific sets of hackers--the "good" and the "bad."

Taking this one step further, without saying so in such

specific words, Bazzell seems to imply that robot developers should hire as many law-abiding hackers as possible.

This way scientists and robotic companies can take pro-active action, plugging potential flaws in programming that nefarious hackers might exploit. In essence, by doing so the creators of robots would position their industry to avoid the types of "flaws and weaknesses" that already have been built into the Internet's infrastructure.

"Many people believe that hackers are these evil misfits that operate individually in dark basements and are motivated by money or a desire to cause unnecessary evil," Bazzell said in the "Forbes" interview. "In reality, hackers are simply very smart people that work in groups to bring change.

"Sometimes they are misguided and inapprorpiate, but they often use their skills to expose hidden details of governments and corporations. Obviously this crosses the line of overexposure often, but most hackers believe that their actions are justified."

Expect Problems Without "Friendly Hackers"

The medical industry, general business and all of society should anticipate significant problems unless robot developers employ hackers as their allies.

Whether or not officials want to acknowledge that the most skilled hackers have an innate ability to think "out of the box," creatively devising ways to infiltrate intended targets. Just as important, another critical factor emerges, namely the fact that the most "successful" hacking teams are methodical in reaching their goals.

Also, another misconception promulgated by the news media and entertainment industry is that hackers work lightning fast in achieving their objectives. To the contrary, doing these high-level individual "jobs" often takes many months or even years. When failure occurs--and it often does--these experts must "start all over again."

Cognizant of these critical factors, hackers working as

allies for robotics companies also need to think of the many creative or unique ways that their devilish counterparts would use when attempting to infiltrate medical robots.

Only by doing this in a consistent and methodical way can robotics companies take significant steps to prevent such intrusions--particularly instances involving medical robots. Otherwise, if flaws are left open for abuse, the healthcare industry and all of society will suffer severe consequences.

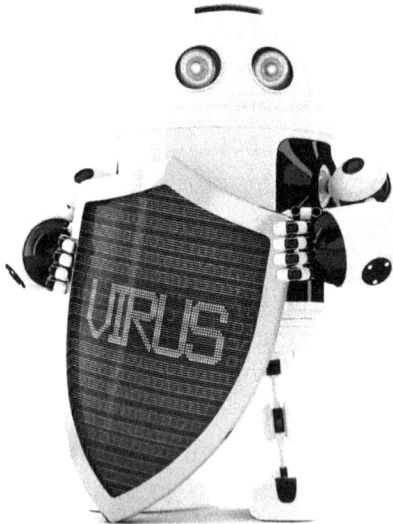

Chapter 27
Artificial Intelligence

Briefly mentioned several times earlier, the success or failure of advanced robots eventually will hinge on whether scientists develop useful Artificial Intelligence.

Often called by the abbreviation "AI," this term designates a human-like intelligence confined within autonomous machines-- independent from people.

This aspect of the robotics industry has emerged as highly controversial; some observers insist that high-level AI will always remain impossible, while others argue otherwise.

As if these factors were not already enough to inflame the issue, some people insist that only God can create viable intelligence. This philosophy contrasts with the theories of scientists who argue that they already have made significant strides in generating high-IQ robots.

Whatever people think or feel about this intensifying issue, there can be no denying that scientists keep moving "full-speed ahead" to develop AI. Their efforts have theoretically begun accelerating as fast as an unstoppable speed train.

Legal or Illegal

So far there have been no formal attempts to criminalize AI-development efforts, which some people insist are "inhuman" and against "the will of God Almighty."

An anonymous conventional, mainstream and allopathic oncologist composed a compelling and riveting essay on this urgent and vital topic; yet his article remains unavailable to the general public. Even so, his well-researched essay proves that AI lacks the unique and God-given ability that humans have to analyze data and also to have "rational thought."

While increasing numbers of electrical engineers insist otherwise, the development of AI strikes at the very core of what life means to many people.

Will this issue ultimately pit people with liberal ideologies against conservatives? Will atheists who refuse to believe in God enter legal battles against religious organizations insist mankind should never create "fake intelligence?"

The previously mentioned controversy of RoboSex is likely to create additional fury within the legal industry. This aspect becomes urgent, particularly if AI enables people to engage in intimate physical intimacy with machines; such interactions would accurately mimic the human-to-human experience--which until now has only been dictated by Mother Nature.

Society Lacks Significant Oppositon

During the mid-2010s as robotics and AI development accelerated, society lacked any strong broad-scale efforts to criminalize or ban such scientific advancements.

At that pivotal juncture, researchers and scientists kept moving forward with their various tests and new technologies for fine-tuning Artificial Intelligence. Robotics company executives predicted that AI would eventually have two primary platforms:

Robotics: As stated earlier, AI would be used by advanced robots.

Computer-based applications: These would be used by numerous industries, such as the previously mentioned automatic-writing applications, systems designed to replace financial advisors, accounting, and many other types of applications.

The non-stop race to put AI into use reached a fever pitch by the dawn of 2016, when the news media released daily news stories on these efforts.

In a one-week period, for instance, numerous major multi-billion-dollar international corporations made separate announcements; each firm had just started to use or develop its own independent AI system. These firms, many traded on major stock exchanges, ranged from Accenture and Facebook, to Google and its partnet company, Alphabet.

216

Sizzling Allegations Emerged

Liberal and conservative publications during the same week took different spins on the issue.

"Artificial Intelligence could be the next big revolution to impact society and increase social inequality in the next 20 years," said a "Huffington Post" article. "The increasing ability for intelligent computers to comprehend tasks means that robots could take over a third of our jobs in the next 20 years."

The Huffington story quoted an article in the "Guardian," which chronicled a 300-page study concluding that AI will eventually exacerbate social inequality within individual communities.

The study by Bank of America and Meryl Lynch compared the advent of AI to the steam and electronic evolutions that each transformed the global economy.

"We are facing a paradigm shift which will change the way we live and work," the report said. "The pace of disruptive technological innovation has gone from linear to parabolic in recent years. Penetration of robots and Artificial Intelligence has hit every industry sector, and has become an integral part of our everyday lives."

The "Great Race of AI"

Streams of car manufacturers including Toyota suddenly joined the race into the Artificial Intelligence realm by late 2015.

The "arms race" and the "space race" among nations from the mid-1900s had been replaced by efforts of many kinds of corporations to enter this new type of competetion.

Theoretically, the so-called "losers" who failed to develop high-level AI systems would be left penniless. International companies and super-power nations began to realize that they would get left behind without such technology.

On a technical level, scientists classify AI as "the study and design of intelligent agents," according to a wide variety of research articles, magazine stories and textbooks. These systems strive to achieve pre-defined goals by first perceiving their environments.

As far back as 1955, researchers strived to launch the initial AI technologies, when John McCarthy--a computer expert and cognitive scientist, became the first person to coin the phrase "Artificial Intelligence."

An Ultimate Challenge

Scientists have been plagued by persistent, nagging challenges in this overall effort since the efforts to develop workable AI systems began accelerating in the 1970s.

Researchers have persistently been bogged down in their ongoing efforts to effectively make the various subsystems of machines that communicate with each other.

Part of this difficulty stems from the unchangable fact that the many AI researchers worldwide grew up or were trained in vastly different cultures.

The world's many diverse societies have various technical, moral and value systems, as previosuly mentioned. These factors, in turn, have increased the difficulties in universally reaching solutions to problems, so-called "fixes that everyone can agree upon."

Massive, highly technical and mathematics-based textbooks and scientific reports have been written on the subject. These intermixed systems are often far too complex for even super-intelligent people to fully understand.

Know the Basics

People interested in the healthcare industry and a wide variety of other business sectors need to have an easy-to-understand basic knowledge of AI technology. In summary, here are the essential platforms that scientists are trying to maximize:

General Intelligence: This is the basic long-term goal, a general knowledge base within individual AI systems. This would give all high-level AI machines the necessary information required to address, solve or perform specific tasks.

Reasoning: Robots or computer-based systems supported by AI would never be "workable" or "fully functional," unless the systems have effective logic that helps them accurately identify objects--before applying all essential data to make decisions.

Morals and values: These previously mentioned critical factors play a significant role in the ultimate choices made by AI systems. Such conclusions are often a "matter of opinion," and therefore must be pre-programmed into the systems.

Planning: Similar to the way that human beings do, in order to be fully effective robots or computer-based systems must have the ability to recognize problems and to "envision goals"--before using all available data to carry out an effective plan.

Learning: Far more effective than "mere humans," the superior AI systems must have the abilities to: collect information in order to "learn," self-teach lessons based on past "mistakes;" and amid this process determine the safest and most effective tasks.

Natural language processing: Instantly, naturally and effectively speak or somehow communicate vital information, using all the many known human languages--plus all the various essential computer coding systems as well.

Perception is the Key

Humans and many other types of animals have a keen ability of "perception," the process of accurately sensing things without necessarily being "told the answers."

Without machines, in nature this involves an instinctive, vital and urgent need for animals to survive and to safely adapt to continually changing environments.

This is why some animals have a keen sense of smell, identifying potential food or enemies--in some instances from great distances. The senses of hearing, sight, touch, and temperature are among factors that help animals including humans get the information or answers that they need--data necessary for survival.

Additionally, many humans possess a unique ability to perceive whether another individual is worried or happy--or perhaps lying or telling the truth. This involves slight nuances or changes in facial expressions, vocal inflections or body languages.

Signs such as these are particularly vital to doctors amid their patient evaluations. Physicians are taught to generate their medical prognosis based on known data; these medical professionals often use their perceived observations, "perceptions and intuitive abilities" when reaching a medical diagnosis.

AI Challenges the Healthcare Industry

All the various highly complex and interlinked challenges in developing effective AI systems will have an increasingly strong impact on health care.

Besides being a matter of life and death, decisions made by human doctors can significantly impact an individual patient's long-term quality of life.

All along, many cultures worldwide have vastly different medical treatment methods--plus a significant array of moral and value systems, as previously mentioned.

Thus, a robot and its accompanying AI system developed to treat a typical U.S.-born, fourth-generation American would likely have a vastly different treatment protocol than such machines built to treat patients from undeveloped countries.

Such diverging factors are among the many legitimate reasons why any effort to build a universally accepted, viable and effective robot-AI mix seems unlikely--if not impossible. Failure in this regard could cause patients far more harm than good.

Massive Amounts of Data Involved

With AI as a core component, medical industry robots and machines serving other industries will require massive amounts of data to "make decisions" and perform tasks. These criteria would be required of high-level, high-performance robots or computer systems that process and use information in various ways. Among them:

Stastical methods: In an effort to produce the best results, AI-enhanced and autonomous robots will use all known data to compute and analyze the various optional tasks or methods. Critics have complained that such strategies are far too focused, possibly leading to problems.

Computational intelligence: Sometimes called "soft computing," this method strives to use artificial neural networks that simulate actual biological conditions. This system melds "machine learning" with the actual makeup of living organisms. When effective, this would mirror the functions and sensational processing speed of the human brain.

Traditional Symbolic AI: Since the beginning of the modern AI-development efforts in the mid-1950s, scientists have strived to develop a "symbol system" to help machines accurately process information. This would be somewhat--or significantly--different from the systems that are based on actual living organisms.

Ultimately, when considering all these various and diverging methods of collecting and processing data, at least one thing becomes clear: "Scientists face a formidable challenge in developing universally effective, automonous medical robots."

Accepting AI in Medical Robots

An interntionally acclaimed vice president of a global company has identified at least five areas of the healthcare industry that would benefit from Artificial Intelligence, according to an October 2015 article in "International Business Times." The article quoted Eugene Borukhovich of SoftServe as listing these benefits:

Drug responses: Patients have different responses to a specific type of chemotherapy drugs. A report cited by Borukhovich indiciates that AI could enable doctors to predict which patients using the drug Paclitaxel would experience improvements.

Start-up uses: A new company, AiCure, was already benefitting from a mobile phone app system used by patients, a process desgined to confirm whether these people have taken prescription medications.

Wearable robots: According to a Microsoft developer, the previosuly mentioned and growing industry of wearable robots is being enhanced to monitor the biometrics of people using the devices. Researchers are using "smart algorithms" that are still under development, in order to "know about the user and his or her biometrics in a steady state to recognize patterns and opportunities to improve the owner's heatlh and fitness."

Alzheimer's Patients: The Department of Computer Science at the University of Washington has been using AI in an effort to improve the quality of life and enhance the independence of Alzheimer's patients.

Smarter drug development: A previously mentioned computer platform, the "IBM Watson," has been working with various drug companies in analyzing massive amounts of data in order to "visualize the relationship between drugs and other potential ailments."

Extensive Challenges Remain

While the various AI systems just mentioned seem promising, at least as of 2015 scientists still had a long way to go in developing an effective, and usuable autonomous and universally accepted Artificial Intelligence system for the medical industry.

Daniela Hernandez of "Kaiser Health News" admitted that AI remained in "an infant stage of development."

Yet scientists continually reported that they expected significant advancements within the critical AI segment of the robotics and computer-based data industries.

Amid these ongoing efforts, some doctors including a Long Island dermatologist Kavita Mariwalla reported that they had successfully used AI systems to identify, find and obtain rarely used drugs to effectively treat specific ailments.

"AI and robots excel at following pre-set rules," said an

article in "The Guardian." "People will thrive when they learn to harness machines for data insights, which they can use for problem-solving and innovation. An architect, for example, will be able to work much faster than today because of the range of technologies available, such as augmented reality visualization and virtual reality headsets. But providing a solution that fits within the constraints of space, planning restrictions, budget and aesthetic would be nigh-on impossible to automate."

Are Caring and Empathetic AI "Personalities" Possible?

As just about everyone knows, doctors earn reputations for having "good," bad," or "merely acceptable" bedside manners.

These terms supposedly describe the person's perceived personality, specifically the apparent ability to genuinely empathize and care for patients. Typical people often consider a good bedside manner as essential in their doctors, particularly the ability to effectively communicate and listen to concerns.

Such attributes are so important to patients that when they proclaim this is a "good doctor" or a "bad doctor," the people are referring specifically to a particular doctor-and-patient relationship.

Cognizant of these critical factors, scientists and electrical engineers face a formidable challenge when striving to develop effective, likeable and empathetic "RoboDoctors." A superior machine not only would need to have the intuitive ability to sense a patient's fears or true desires, but the device also would need to interact with the person in a manner perceived as "truly human."

Imagine a patient who becomes angry, afraid or confused upon gettting a sense that the essential communication and interaction is merely with "nuts, bolts and wires." Such a scenario emerges as disturbing, particularly when taking into account that the person's survival would hinge on "decisions" and actions made by high-level robots.

RoboDoctors that Behave like Jerks?

Amazingly, scientists have been developing robots and AI systems that behave at least a bit like "jerks," a sassy and spicy behavior somewhat akin to humans.

At least according to an "Inverse" article, scientists are programming AI this way because salty or cutting-edge artificial personalities seem much more believable to people. This contrasts with robots that are always hand-holding or teary-eyed with sullen, drawn and overly empathetic expressions.

The article quoted an IBM Labs computer scientist, David Konopnicki, who insisted that in order to emerge as believable and effective, AI must be designed to fulfill the user's expectations amid one-on-one interactions with the machines. Konopnicki specializes in "affective computing," a specialized branch of computer science where the machine picks up on clues from a person's individual characteristics.

The person's signals range from hand movements to facial gestures and vocal inflection. Immediately after collecting this data, a "sassy robot" could interact with the person in a way that seems much more believable. Studies consistently show that people report having a better experience with robots that detect emotion and extract empathy.

"We might not consciously expect our robots to be able to emote and empahtize the way we do, but research shows that we respond better to robots that do," the "Inverse" article said. "Even if you know you're chatting with a computer, you expect the same approach. You want the system to address your informational needs, as well as your emotional needs."

Mainstream Media Ignored this Critical Story

Shockingly, the mainstream media has generally ignored the accelerating advancements in AI technology.

"This is the opposite of the famed Boy-Who-Cried-Wolf situation," some observers might say. "There is just as much danger in remaining ignorant, than society faces when overreacting to such situations."

By November 2015, news articles on AI developments appeared at a steady daily pace, although these details rarely made headlines in mainstream newspapers or primary TV news programs.

Yet anyone searching for these specific details online found a proverbial goldmine of updated information and new developments.

Yes, there were occasional mentions in the mainstream news, as if details were a mere novelty. Yet somehow, rather than becoming increasingly energized by AI advancements, society seemed fixated on what presidential candidates said about their opponents' clothing styles or appearance.

Focus on the "Right Things"

Oblivious to these rapid technology changes that were about to face them, the vast majority of people seemed obsessed with social media and text messaging.

Perhaps most disturbing, a huge percentage of doctors, nurses and other medical professionals remained oblivious to the new AI and robotics systems; the technology was collectively about to "change the entire landscape of the healthcare industry."

During the first week of November, the many separate news stories about Google's AI efforts never got a single mention in the mainstream media. With little fanfare, this company started to:

Freebies: Give AI technologies away for free, so that robotics developers would use the systems in their new machines. If effective as planned, this strategy would give the company a long-term advantage as engineers increasingly began to rely on the technology.

Bait: Advanced and amateur robotics workers and hobbyists quickly began to grab the free Google TensorFlow AI software. This enabled these entrepreneurs to escape high AI acquisition and development prices charged elsewhere, while remaining on the cutting edge of development.

Consumer advantages: According to "TechWorld," an advanced machine-learning engine "has been used by Google to improve speech recognition in the official Google App, as well as forming the image search now available in Google photos."

Consumer dependence: As steadily increasing numbers of entrepreneurs and companies begin to rely on the technology, will Google begin to benefit financially--if and when the corporation starts charging fees for necessary future add-on software?

The First Digital Hospital Opens

These various rapid accelerations in AI came right after the first fully digitalized hospital in North America opened in Toronto, Canada.

"Tech Times" reported that the Humber River Hospital's many advanced software and AI-based services ranged from robot servants to patient touchpads.

Once again the mainstream news media generally ignored this significant story, as a huge percengage of doctors and other medical professionals remained oblivious to these significant changes in medical care.

Like this or not, such changes already were being positioned to rapidly spread throughout the entire medical industry--but only if the digital systems performed as planned.

Among initial digital-based features at the 656-bed Toronto hospital:

Chemotherapy: Instead of using human pharmacists or other people, the facility has robots that mix and prepare drugs as prescribed by physicians. The machines then monitor the dosages given to each cancer patient.

Radiology: Rather than employing human perssonnel for this particular job, the facility uses three robots that position patients during X-ray procedures.

Monitoring: Programmed to track every drug, robots affix bar codes to containers of the pharmceuticals; this is done after the machine prepares and packages the mixtures or compounds. This advanced information technology enabled hospital executives and doctors to accurately monitor medications.

"Hospital hallways and even elevators will be seen with automated robots carrying around medical supplies for the heatlh care team," the "Tech Times" article said. "All hospital beds are equipped with touch pads that patients could use to view their records and medical charts, adjust room temperature according to their liking, make phone calls, play video games, and watch television."

AI Will Increasingly Enter the Mix

If such advancements continued as planned, other hospitals across North America were to adopt similar digital systems-- before or during the spread of AI into the facilities.

In essence, fully digital hospitals serve as the equivalent of chassis and frames of cars. The advent and add-ons of AI will serve as the proverbial motor, enabling the systems to run or move forward--in some instances without direct human assistance.

Three weeks after the Toronto hospital opened, the "Market Watch" financial news service reported that the top open-source, machine-learning AI platform announced the close of its $20 million Series B funding round.

Led by Paxion Capitol Partners, the latest funding effort brought the total collected to $34 million for the company, H2O. ai. While this total might seem a "paltry amount" on the wide scale of international business, some robotics experts viewed this development as significant.

"I'd be shocked if every company in the world wouldn't benefit from using H2O," the story quoted industry expert Michael Marks as saying. "Market Watch" reported that Marks had previously helped build phenomenal growth at companies like Zappos, also transforming Flextronics into a multi-billion-dollar company.

Advances Continued Despite Warnings

The non-stop advances in AI continued at a ferocious pace in health care and other industries, despite warnings from such luminaries as physicist Stephen Hawking, who said: "Computers will overtake humans with AI at some point within the next 100 years."

Despite such dire forecasts, a growing cadre of entrepreneurs, governments and corporations moved full-throttle in efforts to fine-tune and improve AI.

The "Gov Insider" publication quoted Doctor Andy Chun, an associate professor at City University of Hong Kong, as saying that AI involves any software that performs tasks that previously had been uniquely associated with human capabilities.

According to the article, this could range from inate human behavior like seeing and talking, to far more complex tasks like "designing a bridge or diagnosing a patient."

Delving into what many observers including experienced human doctors would consider as extremely dangerous, the article also quotes Chun as saying that governments could use AI systems in highly regulated industries like health care and public safety.

Disturbing Trends Quickly Emerged

As if all these various previously mentioned factors were not already enough to cause ample reason for concern, additional news reports in a wide variety of publications described how scientists attempted to use AI to manipulate human behavior. Among these many instances:

Influencing Humans: According to "PC World," researchers in Singapore began a two-year trial of a smartphone app that attempts to use Artificial Intelligence to influence the "real-world decisions of users."

Satellite Monitoring: According to the "Fast Company" publication, the World Bank had partnered the Orbital Insight firm to have satellites use AI systems for continually monitoring poverty around the world--replacing door-to-door surveys.

Disturbing communications: According to various news reports, millions of young people have started engaging in one-on-one communications with a unique AI system called Xiolace--which uses natural language in voice-initiated chats.

Blind People: According to "International Business Times," scientists at the GiveVision company have developed "augmented reality" software that enables blind people to recognize objects.

Children's Toys: According to a "Washington Post" article published in the "Portland Press Herald," by Christmas of 2015 various companies were making AI-enabled toys for children; the devices answer or respond to specific statements made by the youngsters.

The examples just mentioned are among the many hundreds or even thousands of AI systems that had already entered the consumer marketplace or were well on the way to being introduced to society.

Extensive Dangers Loomed

The rocket-fast rollout of AI into society likely posed extreme dangers, perhaps even to some healthcare applications.

On the surface of this issue was the fact that people readily began to accept these technologies, in most or all instances "putting all their faith and trust" in the systems.

Yet in all likelihood, consumers lacked any notion of who built the devices, let alone how or why these systems were made. In this sense, critics might argue that typical humans willingly allowed themselves to become "as if mere chimpanzees."

The worry here stemmed from the fact that some manufacturers might fail to fully test AI systems. Remember that as previously mentioned some of these technologies might have pre-programmed "moral and value" systems; such characteristics might finally become apparent many months or even years after people purchase them.

When and if such flaws or pre-planned transitions occur,

would consumers or robotics experts still have the necessary time to reverse or correct the adverse situations--such as a computer that begins jabbering about unwanted religious beliefs?

As the age-old saying goes, "only time will tell," particularly within the realm of the healthcare industry.

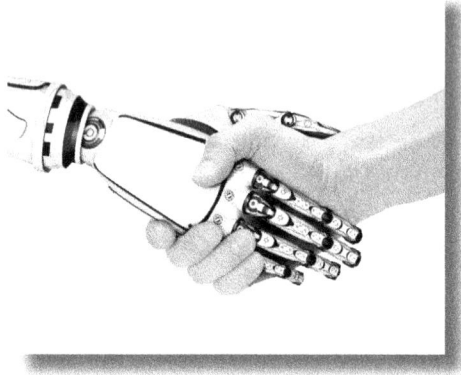

Chapter 28
Medical Robotics Companies Increase

The number of robotics companies specializing in the healthcare industry--or with subsidiaries serving that business sector--began a steady increase in the 2010s.

"The proverbial floodgates have opened in this regard," I tell patients. "We should expect even more increases at a steady pace through the 2020s and beyond."

Among medical robotics companies that have been receiving some of the greatest attention, particularly among doctors and healthcare facility administrators:

Barrett Technology: Initially part of the Massachusetts Institute of Technology, in 1990 this firm spun-off from that institution's Artifical Intelligence Laboratory. The company specializes in the development and design of robotic manipulators. Among its many products are WAM Arms that help senior citizens and infirmed people put on clothes. Engineers have programmed the devices to "learn" how to clothe individual people. Website: *Barrett.com*

Cyberdyne Inc.: Based in Japan, this company with a laboratory at the University of Tsukuba specializes in making and commercializing inventions that "enable and/or augments human motor function by reading nerve signals through the skin," according to a report in "Robotics Business Review." Website: *Cyberdyne.jp/English*

Ekso Bionics: Formerly called Berkeley Bionics, this Richmond, California-based firm, specializes in robotics exoskeletons designed to improve and assist the mobility of disabled people including former soldiers injured in combat. Since being founded in 2005, the firm has formed alliances with major institutions including the University of California in Berkeley. Ekso Bionics has licensed technology with Lockheed Martin Corporation, also receiving grants from the U.S. Department of Defense. The firm licensed products to a major prosthetics company, Ottobock, which will use Ekso technology to generate microprocessor-controlled innovations for prosthetic knees. Website: *EksoBionics.com*

GaitTronics: Within three years after being founded in 2012, this Canadian firm became a spin-off from Carleton University's Advanced Biomechatronics and Locomotion Laboratory. The Ottawa-based firm has used specialized robotics platforms in developing unique expertise for the creation and development of rehabilitation robotics. The spin-off process enabled the company to commercialize a unique robotic product, SoloWalk(tm), that helps caregivers mobilize frail patients at long-term care and acute care facilities. The company says the product enables a greater proportion of patients to become mobile earlier than they would without the devices. Medical experts say that "getting a frail patient to walk can improve clinical outcomes and reduce their length-of-stay in the hospital." Website: *GaitTronics. com*

Hansen Medical: Based in Mountain View, California, the company's robotics specialize in the stable control, manipulation, and accurate positioning of catheters and catheter-based technologies. Website: *HansenMedical.com*

Harmonic Drive, LLC: Based in Peabody, Massachusetts, this company manufactures and designs gearheads and gear component sets. The firm works with companies of all sizes and industry-leading customers; Harmonic Drive serves, in several market segments including medical and assistive, plus military and defense, industrial automation and energy. Website: *HarmonicDrive.net*

Health Robotics: This Italy-based firm founded in 2006 is a leading supplier of robotic-based technology and clinical software automation solutions. The firm is a leading supplier of life-critical intravenous medication automation. More than 250 hospitals on five continents use the company's technology. The company has reported that its unique solutions simultaneously reduce costs, while improving patient safety. Website: *Health-Robotics.com*

Hocoma: This Switzerland-based firm specializes in the medical and assistive industries. The company has been hailed as a global market leader in the development, manufacturing and marketing of robotic and sensor-based devices for functional movement therapy. Website: *Hocoma.com*

Honda Robotics: This Tokyo-based division of Honda Motor Co., Ltd., has subcompanies that specialize in the medical and assistive industries, plus the development of humanoid robots and software. According to various published reports, robotic exoskeletons developed by Honda have a variety of uses ranging from life-changing healthcare assistance machines to military robots. Website: *Honda.com*

Hundai Heavy Industries Co., Ltd.: World-famous for a wide variety of machines and transporation devices ranging from ships to military equipment, this South Korea-based company has various branches that now include medical and assistive. According to news reports, Hyundai has developed a partnership that will build surgical robots. In 2012, the company announced that it had opened a laboratory "dedicated to building surgery robots within the Asian Institute of Life Sciences." Website: *english.hhi.co.kr*

Innovation Associates: This Johnson City, New York-based company specializes in the healthcare and medical-assistive industries. The firm works with hospitals and governments while developing pharmacy automation technologies. The U.S. Navy has awarded a multi-million-dollar contract to the company. Website: *Innovat.com*

InTouch Health: This Santa Barbara, California-based company is a leading innovator of robots that enable doctors to communicate with patients in hospitals. Industry experts categorize this firm as a leading provider of the Telehealth Network and Services. Touted as delivering "high-quality virtual care, any time and anywhere," the firm has helped more than 110 healthcare systems deploy Telehealth programs. Features include TV-like screens that enable patients to see real-time images of their doctor, while the physician also can view an image of the person. The overall system is designed to seamlessly and quickly use its "industry leading combination of professionals, processes and practices." Besides healthcare and medical-assistive, the company also specializes in the mobile and "telepresence" industries. Website: *InTouchHealth.com*

Intuitive Surgical: This Sunnyvale, California-based company has gained a positive reputation for marketing, manufacturing and designing da Vinci surgical systems. The company has designed a variety of surgical services that range from head and neck surgeries, to procedures that include urologic, gynecologic, cardiothoracic and general medicine. The da Vinci surgical system features include proprietary "wristed" instruments, a 3-D vision system, a patient side-cart and a console or consoles for surgeons. Website: *IntuitiveSurgical.com*

Kinova Robotics: Based in Quebec, this robotics company--hailed as one of Canada's fastest-growing firms--specializes in the healthcare and medical-assistive industries, plus service robots and manipulators. The company says that its assistive robotics empowers disabled people to push beyond their current boundaries and limitations. Website: *KinovaRobotics.com*

MAKO Surgical: With offices in Fort Lauderdale, Florida, this medical device company markets robotic arm solutions and orthopedic implants worldwide. A primary product is MAKOplasty, "a restorative surgical solution that enables orthopedic surgeons to treat patient-specific osteoarthritic disease." According to news reports, the company's RIO Robotic Arm Interactive Orthopedic System supports a "surgeon's ability to more accurately align and position a hip implant." According to published reports, in 2013 Stryker bought MAKO for $1.65 billion. Website: *MakoSurgical.com*

Maxon Precision Motors, Inc.: This Fall River, Massachusetts-based company specializes in healthcare and medical-assistive devices, plus a wide variety of other industries. Besides airborne applications and education-research, these business sectors range from industrial automation, maritime, military defense, mining exploration, and others. Among its most famous devices is the Philae Robot Space Probe, which landed on Comet 67P--marking the first time a manmade device successfully touched down on a comet. Way back in 2009, the company's microdrives were certified for implantation in people. Website: *MaxonMotorUSA.com*

Medrobotics Corporation: Formerly Cardiorobotics, Inc., this Massachusetts-based company specializes in creating multi-linked robotic technology for surgical procedures. Website: *Medrobotics.com*

Open Bionics: Based at the University of the West of England on the Frenchay Campus in Bristol, this company specializes in making accessible and affordable robotic prosthetic hands. Website: *OpenBionics.com*

Ottobock: With offices in Germany, this company serves as a global leader in prosthetic orthotic medical devices. Serving mobility challenges worldwide, the firm has more than 6,000 employees working in at least 49 branch facilities. Website: *Ottobock.de*

Panasonic: Based in Osaka, Japan, this company formerly known as Matsushite Electric Industrial Co., Ltd., specializes in the medical-assistive industry, plus industrial automation and mobile service robots. The company develops, manufactures and sells electronic products worldwide. According to news reports, Panasonic's Blue Collar Delivery Robots have been making gains in U.S. Hospitals. In 2014, the company released a lineup of medical products, leading at least one industry analyst to conclude that "it would be easy to annoint the company as the uncontested owner of the automated healthcare crown." Also that year, Panasonic launched its new corporate brand slogan: "A Better Life, A Better World." Website: *Panasonic.net*

Restoration Robotics: This Mountainview, California-based company founded in 2002 develops and offers robotic surgery systems for hair transplants. Website: *RRobotics.com*

SRI International: This Menlo Park, California-based company hailed as a leader in research and development has been credited with creating various new industries. The company specializes in healthcare and medical-assistive, plus agriculture, and miltiary defense security, plus the supply-chain and retail industries. According to published reports, the company delivers state-of-the-art robotics to the commercial and governmental markets. SRI reports that "our robotics teams invent, apply and commercialize components, software and systems that are redefining the robot revolution." SRI's many medical and surgical devices include dexterous surgical tools, devices serving the pediatric market, compact chemical and bioligical sensor development, biosensors, digital X-ray systems, and advanced materials for devices such as hearing aids. Website: *SRI.com*

Swisslog: This Switzerland-based company specializes in providing integrated logistics solutions for hospitals, distribution centers and warehouses. Along with its competitors including Aethon, Panasonic and Vecna, the company has been instrumental in providing blue collar delivery robotic systems in hospitals. In 2014, Swisslog acquired FORTE Industries for $335 million, giving the firm access to advanced mobile robotics. Website: *Swisslog.com*

SynTouch LLC: This Los Angeles-based company specializes in the medical-assistive and automation industries. SynTouch develops technolgoy that gives robots the ability to replicate the human sense of touch. The company reports that its lead product, BioTac, mimics physical properties and sensory capabilities of the human fingertip. Website: *SynTouchLLC.com*

Touch Bionics Limited: With offices in the United Kingdom, this company specializes in the healthcare, medical-assistive, and service robot industries. According to news reports, the company has been instrumental in developing bionic hands and bionic fingers. Some robotics industry observers believe these technologies or applications could be instrumental in developing advanced humanoid robots. The company has successfully attached these non-surgical devices to the limbs of patients. Website: *TouchBionics.com*

Vecna Technologies: Like the previously mentioned Aethon, Panasonic and Swisslog businesses, this Cambridge, Massachusetts-based company plays an instrumental role in the development of delivery robots used by hospitals. Website: *Vecna. com*

VGo Communications: Besides healthcare and medical-assitive, this Nashua, New Hampshire-based company also serves the mobile telepresence and education-research industries. According to a July 2015 article in "Robotics Business Review," VGo formalized what had been a 10-year relationship with the previously mentioned Vecna Technologies. Website: *VGoCom.com*

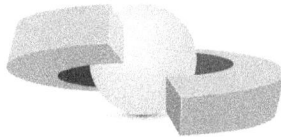

Medical Robotics Companies

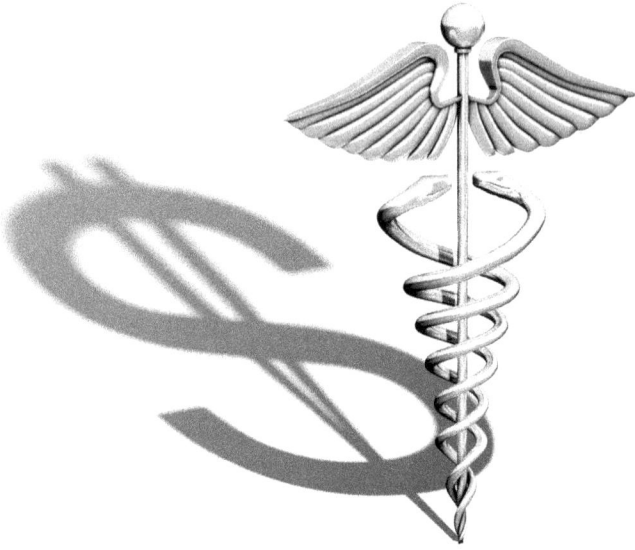

Chapter 29
Will Patient Costs Skyrocket?

Many analysts expect extensive growth throughout the medical robotics sector, while the previously mentioned companies and additional non-medical firms help lead the way.

Keep in mind that the aforementioned companies comprise only a small percentage of such ventures, which keep being lauched or continue growing at a steady pace.

Besides the continually increasing rate of technolgical discoveries, the growth of the specialized robotics sector will hinge largely on the willingness of hospital and clinic administrators to accept new and unique robotics or AI-based systems.

Will the roll-out and advent of these systems ultimately increase or drive down the overall cost of healthcare? At least into the late 2010s, such questions remained unanswered. Yet some experts anticipated that patient fees would sharply increase as a result.

"In every industry but one, technology makes things better and cheaper," said a 2013 "MIT Technology Review" article. "Why is it that innovation increases the cost of health care?"

Compelling Arguments Erupted

The MIT article's author, Jonathan S. Skinner, argued that with increasing intensity some observers have predicted an "armageddon" in the rise of health care costs--plus what he said would emerge as the inescapable bankruptcy of Medicare.

Many analysts insist that technology fails to generate inflation in other sectors of the economy; the experts seem to agree that technological advancements in the medical industry are already increasing costs within that business sector. These developments reportedly are among factors that require U.S.

consumers to pay more per capita on healthcare than in any other country.

Complicating matters on a tragic level, there still seemed to be no consensus on whether the advent of robotics and AI would sharply increase U.S. patient fees.

Some observers blame what they call a complex or dizzying array of new medical treatments and methods. Numerous systems provide tremendous value per patient dollar spent, while other technolgies fail to provide cost benefits.

The proverbial and unwanted "poison pill" in this regard comes from health insurance companies, which overall have been willing to pay for most types of treatments--in some instances whether or not those protocols emerge as effective.

Lacking Scientific Evidence

At least from the view of some healthcare industry analysts, the surging medical fees stem at least partly from new and relatively unproven medical technologies. The worst of these supposed advancements lack scientific evidence to prove they are effective treatments.

Adding to these woes, in some instances hospitals and clinics eager to remain competitive eagerly buy many of these highly expensive--yet unproven--devices.

In keeping with standard or conventional business practices, these costs are passed on to the patients, primarily through expensive monthly health insurance premiums. These expenses can reach offensively high levels.

The "big losers" here are consumers, who get stuck with ludricious "over-the-moon" fees passed on to them in the form of skyrocketing insurance premiums.

Worsening matters multi-fold, as previously mentioned, Obamacare--which many consumers are now calling "the Unaffordable Health Care Act"--requires all U.S. citizens to buy these weak, overly expensive and complicated policies. The big winners here are insurance companies and inept government bureaucrats, while typical consumers emerge as the Big Losers.

Tragic Outcome Became Obvious

During the week after President Barack Obama was first elected into office in 2008, I went into "mourning." Like many other physicians I saw the proverbial writing on the wall, the fact that Obama's over-the-top socialist policies would wreak havoc on the entire medical industry.

Like many Americans, I know good, hard-working people who can no longer visit a doctor due to Obamacare. Adding insult to injury, at least one industrious person that I know was even "kicked out of Obamacare" due to absolutely no fault of his own.

Infecting these proverbial wounds even more, unless someone can prove otherwise I predict that the Rise of the Robots throughout the medical industry will cause health care costs to skyrocket to even more "maddening levels" in the United States and worldwide.

When that happens, healthcare services might improve somewhat, and even become more efficient in many instances. However, if patient fees surge upward as I predict due to robotics, the number of people able to benefit will sharply decrease.

As if to thumb their noses at the general public, as previously mentioned all politicians seemed oblivious to the surge in medical robotics. This disturbing factor essentially sets the stage for more widespread tragedy throughout the healthcare industry.

Expect an Adverse "Ripple Affect"

Put together as a whole, these various factors could very well destroy the American and world economies. Yes, Obamacare is a steadily worsening self-destructive time bomb, poised to make the entire economy implode. We are talking in terms of a multi-trillion-dollar negative impact.

The increasingly rapid spread of robotics into the entire medical industry will accelerate to extreme levels. But does this mean that robotics companies and medical industry administrators should suddenly stop all efforts to create and distribute such machines?

To the contrary, entrepreneurs and burgeoning robotics companies should continue developing effective non-robotic devices, as long as three factors become priorities:

Ban Obamacare: The entire Obamacare system should be shut down for good, particularly because most Americans want this treacherous system obliterated.

Get Results: Focus on developing robotics systems that get proven and positive results, including a lowering of personnel costs--ultimately reducing consumer fees.

Criminalize AI: Criminalize any medical robotics system that uses autonomous machines designed to replace human doctors and nurses.

Only by taking these sensible and logical actions now, relatively early in the development of medical robotics, can authorities control the situation. Otherwise the medical industry and healthcare costs likely will spiral out of control.

Expect Tragic Outcomes

Each of the various and necessary solutions just mentioned are unlikely to occur, for a variety of economic and political reasons.

As a result, typical citizens throughout the United States should expect an "economic armageddon" to erupt in every business sector.

Many people say that during the first 15 years of the 21st Century the world became increasingly dangerous in almost every regard. The countless technological advances became far too complex and intermixed for most people to understand.

On the flip side, the administrators of large hospitals in recent years have seriously been considering the addition of new robotics technologies; this is done partly to increase profit--while decreasing or even eliminating employee expenses.

Meantime, however, even by 2010, advancements in

surgical robotics had sharply increased patient costs, at least according to various reports by medical industry experts.

Disturbing Truths Emerged

According to a research article published in the "New England Journal of Medicine" as the 2010s began, health care costs had already increased by at least $2.5 billion as a direct result of new robotic surgery technologies.

Over a relatively short period just prior to then the number of such surgeries annually had skyrocketed to 205,000, up from just 80,000 procedures a short time before. The costs and number of surgeries likely have surged since then due to robots.

The big lure attracting doctors and patients came from the fact that robotic surgeries are relativley fast, causing little pain and with quick recovery times for patients.

These factors have failed to alleviate the legitimate concerns of numerous industry observers, who insist that some robotic surgeries are done unnecessarily--thereby increasing overall patient costs.

"In addition to costs, there are other concerns with robotic surgeries," David Lipschitz said in his "Lifelong Health" article. "While it has opened up complex and very difficult surgeries to minimally invasive approaches, the system is often used for operations such as gallbladder surgery and hysterectomies, which could just as easily be performed using cheaper endoscopic approaches."

Demand Surged

The demand and use of robotic surgeries started increasing significantly early in the 21st Century, almost as soon as these technologies became available.

The advent of such new systems seemed to generate a philosophy that "if we have got this new technology, we might as well use it."

These various factors bring forth the prospect of even more

potentially disturbing changes throughout the medical industry. Among the obvious questions that should continue to arise:

Unnecessary systems: Will the race to overtake competition in healthcare entice some hospitals and clinics to adopt certain unnecessary and expensive robotics systems?

Ripple effect: Will these enticements spark a dangerous "medical industry" race, where hospitals and clinics spend far too much on unproven robotics systems in an effort to "be the best" or to remain competitive?

Unstoppable competition: Will such a whirlpool of competition reach an "unstoppable level," where medical businesses fear that they will be overcome, unless those ventures spend huge amounts for unproven robotics?

If the past is any indication of future outcomes, in all likelihood most medical facilities will embrace the latest robotics syetems--often as soon as such technology becomes available. Such a "keep-up-with-the-Joneses" business strategy likely would cause great financial hardship for typical consumers, while increasing the already cumbersome levels of confusion throughout the health insurance industry.

Potential Positive Business Outcomes

Intermixed with the various negative possibilities comes the suggestion by some robotics industry experts that these machines actually will improve efficiency--while reducing overall costs.

In a July 2014 article, "HFM Magazine" predicted that the demand for medical robots will surge "exponentially" because of the many advantages the machines offer.

According to proponents of such devices, the story said, "robots can curtail labor costs, add operational efficiencies, increase precision, create better clinical outcomes, and replace humans in potentially unsafe situations.

"But these systems are not one-size-fits-all and health facility professionals need to be part of a careful and deliberative team-based process--to make the right decisions regarding selection, technology maturity, logistics, infrastructure planning and maintenance."

To do this effectively, the article said, operators of these facilities need to use machines other than just surgical robots; administrators also should consider the many additional types of machines used by hospitals. These range from robots that handle linens and trash, to devices that collect, prepare, transport, analyze and store laboratory samples--plus many more duties.

Ultimalty this overall analytical process would involve an in-depth cost analysis. The various criteria would range from the length of patient stays and the percentage of re-admissions, to whether staffers and patients accept such devices.

Cost Considerations Become Increasingly Complex

Besides the many types of medical robots already mentioned, according to various published reports the various additional machines subject to cost analysis include:

Autonomous Mobile Transport Robots: These include "automated guided vehicles" or AVGs, that deliver a wide varity of materials throughout hospitals. Some AVGs are so specialized that they need fully dedicated hallways and elevators. Hospitals and clinics need to integrate the expenses of building these infrastructures into their cost analysis. Some AVGs feature pre-installed Wi-Fi systems that enable people to continually monitor these devices. Officials also need to consider the cost of building and maintaining docking stations where each AVG gets recharged at least every 10 hours.

Environmental Disinfection Robots: Increasingly popular and undergoing trails by the late 2010s, these previously mentioned machines continually disinfect patient rooms and operating rooms. These robots use either of two disinfection methods, either ultraviolet light (UV) or hydrogen peroxide vapors (HPV.) The UV machines reportedly cost from $104,000 to $124,500 to purchase, or the devices can be obtained via 36-month lease agreements at about $3,000 per month. The HPV robots are much less expensive at $44,000 to $64,000, but when using them the facilities would have the additional cost of sealing ducts and various room openings; this is a requirement in order to prevent the spread of toxic HPV. Once again, the facilities' operators would need to consider the potential cost savings of eliminating certain employees.

Laboratory Robots: These machines perform numerous tasks. Besides preparing and managing specimens in tubes, laboratory robots track the testing process and handle post-analytical storage. These devices perform many additional complex duties. But existing hospital laboratories need to be modified or rebuilt to accommodate the robots; this largely because the machines have mobility functions vastly different from people. Adding to the challenge, laboratory robots also must be integrated with a hospital's existing laboratories and informational (IT) systems. Such expenses also need to be considered in generating any cost-benefit analysis.

Pharmaceutical Robots: A cost-benefit of whether to use the aforementioned pharmaceutical robots is crucial to any hospital or medical clinic, before deciding whether to use these devices. Some of these machines perform tasks within the building's main pharmacy or in a oncology infusion area. These robots are linked to computer-based systems. The many benefits include a reduction or elimination of human exposure to hazardous drugs, plus the administration of precise doses and enhanced productivity. Besides eliminating unwanted particulates from the air, the machines also handle barcoding, automatically manage waste and decrease the likelihood of contamination within the drug-preparation area. The costs of acquiring pharmaceutical robots are high by almost any standard, from $400,000 to $1.5 million. Even so, these machines have the potential to automate up to 90 percent of tasks that typically had been performed by people within hospital pharmacies. Thus, administrators need to analyze cost data, before determining whether transitioning to this system would save money. Overall, costs for buying and using these machines can increase, due to inescapable expenses for maintenance and related work. In addition, the necessary expenses might include potentially significant fees for installing any required Information Technology.

Sterile Processing Robots: These devices remained in early-stage development by early 2016, while some medical industry observers indicated that the initial prototypes appeared promising. Located in a 5-foot square Plexiglas enclosure, these machines perform a huge variety of functions. Besides counting and repacking instruments, Sterile Processing Robots inspect, sort and clean medical equipment. These include precision instruments used by physicians and nurses, devices that need to remain sterile to decrease the likelihood of infection. While all this seemed promising, however, the earliest versions of these machines had difficulty disassembling medical devices that have multiple parts. As with the other healthcare machines, administrators would need to determine whether Sterile Processing Robots would essentially "pay for themselves"--enabling the facilities to eliminate human employees as a cost-saving strategy, while increasing efficiency.

Analysis Becomes Essential

Besides the types of medical robots already suggested for an in-depth cost analysis, numerous additional automated machines also must be considered. This is particularly true among large hospitals that intend or hope to go "fully digital."

The many additional robots or AI systems, some briefly mentioned in earlier chapters or sections, include:

Therapeutical Robots: These help or assist developmentally disabled children, while continually monitoring their progress.

Telepresence Robots: The devices that go throughout the Emergency Room and to various patient rooms, enabling doctors located at other facilities to "remotely visit" patients.

Non-invasive Radiosurgery Robots: Using image-controlled and machine-guided technology systems, they deliver high-energy radiation beams with great precision.

Exoskeleton-powered Robots: These wearable devices strive to reduce the morbidity of paraplegic patients, while augmenting physical therapy.

Daily Care Robots: Assisting disabled people and senior patients, these machines perform daily activities such as serving meals.

Extreme Risks Can Reap Tremendous Rewards

The business risks of integrating robots into a hospital or clinic can be risky, while also potentially generating great rewards in revenue, cost savings and efficiency.

Hospital and clinic administrators need to thoroughly vet the technologies, in order to determine beforehand if robots have a chance for success in their facilities.

Just as assential, these various managers, directors and executives need to implement comprehensive planning. When done the "right way," these changes can occur in a relativley smoothe and hassle-free way.

For that to happen, healthcare industry leaders must initiate well-timed and carefully planned robotics installations.

Simultaneously and with just as much focus, the facilities need to retrain staffers or recruit qualified personnel. Healthcare businesses where administrators continually monitor medical robotics industry changes--and immediately strive to benefit from these technologies--will position their facilities for greater profit than their competitors.

These factors will accelerate an industry-wide "keep-up-with-the-Joneses" philosophy in which facilities without such technologies would no longer be viable. Sadly, these considerations might motivate officials to make decisions too fast--thereby unnecessarily endangering patients.

Helping Patients Remains a Crucial Goal

The steady transition into medical robotics throughout the healthcare industry is more than about saving money, according to the American Society of Mechanical Engineers (ASME).

The organization's publication states that "advocates of robotic surgery, for example, claim the da Vinci surgical robot achieves significantly better outcomes than either radiation or traditional surgery--in delicate procedures such as radical prostatectomy for prostate cancer.

"They say robotic surgery can remove more cancerous tissue with less disruption of adjacent nerve endings than other methods, helping to reduce cancer recurrence and retain sexual function."

For these reasons, the ASME says, by 2012 a whopping 85 percent of patients undergoing prostate cancer surgery selected medical centers offering robotic surgery.

The "New York Times" quoted a Florida surgeon, Vipul Patel, as saying that "From Day One, when I sat down at that robotic console, I knew we would give patients a better outcome. I have not seen anyone who has done a good amount of robotic surgery go back" to the traditional methods.

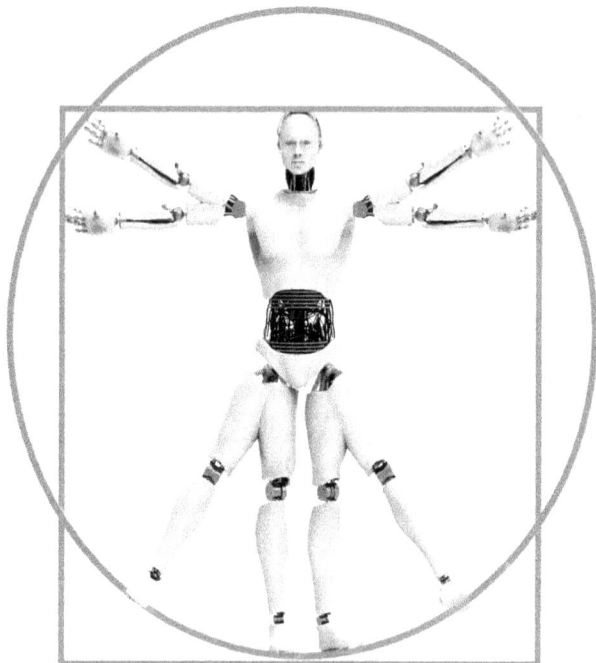

Chapter 30
Essential Robotics History

Who first envisioned robots? Just as essential, when, where and how did initial developments in robotics occur?

The answers to these questions serve as a vital cornerstone of knowledge for anyone eager to learn about medical robotics and other uses for the machines.

The first known in-depth drawings that later would become the primary images of robots were created by the famed inventor and artist Leonardo da Vinci.

This iconic native of Florence, Italy, born out of wedlock, is perhaps best known today as the artist who created such world famous paintings as the Mona Lisa and the Last Supper.

Many people overlook the fascinating fact that da Vinci also became a prolific inventor, sculptor, architect, and mathematician. Insatiably curious, his many interests included general science, music, writing, history, astronomy and geology.

Da Vinci Set the Groundwork

Living from 1452 to 1519, da Vinci's early drawings of robots, helicopters, machine guns, rockets and advanced weaponry became the basis many years later for such devices. Lots of these machines were developed and fine-tuned by entrepreneurs and scientists, primarily during the 19th and 20th Centuries.

Da Vinci's initial conceptual designs became spookily similar to such weapons as the Gatling Gun, tanks, and submarines.

Still hailed today as the ultimate "Renaissance Man," according to historians da Vinci was blessed with an unquenchable curiosity and a "feverishly inventive imagination." Perhaps somewhat ironically, these are the same attributes that today's best robotics experts must have to successfully envision and create high-level robots.

Da Vinci's uncannily accurate early studies of the human body, at least in part, helped serve as the basis for at least some medical knowledge. According to da Vinci's memoirs, in around 1507 or 1508 while in his late 50s he met a man over 100 years old who told him that there was nothing wrong with his body other than weakness.

"And thus," da Vinci wrote, "without any movement or sign of any mishap, he passed from this life. And I dissected him to see the cause of so sweet a death."

The Basis for Robotics

This research became one of at least 30 human dissections that da Vinci performed during his lifetime. His meticulous drawings helped serve as a basis for illustrations of the human body, medical literature and--ultimately, at least to some degree-- toward the modern-day development of humanoid robots.

These illustrations became so instrumental and essential to advancements in art and medical technology that in 2013 officials joined to create an exhibit entitled, "Leonardo da Vinci: "The Mechanics of Man."

These images proved so essential to science that officials displayed da Vinci's drawings alongside modern CT and MRI scans. The display helped emphasize what eventually became known as this man's "far-sighted brilliance."

Da Vinci's legendary art and discoveries served as a primary reason why some thriving robotics companies and entrepreneurs in this field have named their patented robots and certain essential human-like machine parts in his honor.

Many Advancements Built Upon Success

In the more than 570 years since da Vinci's birth, a steady succession of physicians, artists and mechanical engineers built upon and advanced his initial work.

Within the field of robotics, these advancements have

steadily accelerated--with the creation of the world's first actual robot prototype in the 1920s.

Since then, of course, robots have become somewhat legendary within many cultures worldwide.

Throughout most of the 20th Century, the concept of robots often became an essential feature or plotting device in science-fiction literature, movies and TV shows.

The word "robot" actually was invented or coined by a Czech playwright, Karel Čapek, for his 1920 play entitled "Rossum's Universal Robots." The play soon became world-famous, and people worldwide quickly started using the word.

Numerous Discoveries Were Necessary

A wide variety of discoveries were later necessary for the basis of today's robotics. These advancements ranged from findings in physics and mathematics, to metallurgy and even biology. Many of these pivotal developments deserve recognition and praise.

Some of the first significant developments occurred during these pivotal years:

1926: The Westinghouse Corporation intorduced "Televox," which users could turn off and on via various devices connected to the unit's cardboard cutout.

1928: In London at the Model Engineers Society, an annual exhibition, inventor W.H. Richards introduced "Eric," one of the first humanoid robots--featuring 11 electromagnets and an aluminum body of armor. A single 12-volt motor powered the device, operated via voice or remote control, and capable of moving its head and hands.

1928: "Gakutensoku" became the first robot in Japan, built and designed by Makoto Nishimura, a widely acclaimed biologist. Capable of changing its facial expressions thanks to an air pressure mechanism, the robot also moved its hands and head. A bird-shaped robot was perched atop the head of Gakutensoku, which displayed a pensive expression whenever the other device wept.

1939: At that year's New York World's Fair, the Westinghouse Electric Corporation introduced "Elektro," a 265-pound, 7-foot-tall humanoid robot that spoke about 700 words and walked via voice command. The cigarette-smoking gadget delighted crowds by blowing up balloons, while also able to move its arms and head.

1948-49: A significant development in the annals of robot history occurred in Briston at the Burden Neurological Institute where William Grey Walter developed the first robots with electric and autonomous features. The devices were capable of exhibiting complex behaviors. This marked the first time that people had tried with varying degrees of success to simulate the human brain's processes in a machine. Walter emphasized the importance of simulating brain functions purely by using analog electronics.

1954: American inventor George Duvol introduced his creation, "Unimate," a programmable and digitally operated robot--which ultimately has served as the foundation for today's modern robotics industry, according to a 2008 article in the "Society of Manufacturing Engineers."

1960: General Motors purchased the first Unimate from Duvol.

1961: At a plant in Trenton, N.J., General Motors installed the first "Unimate." The machine stacked and lifted hot metal from a die-casting device. Today's robotic industry still uses a programmable and digitally operated robotic arm that Duvol had patented.

1963: The Fuju Yusoki Kogyo Company introduced the first palletizing robot; like Kogyo's original, today's similar devices place stacked products and goods on pallets. Prior to the development and widespread use of such robots, these chores had stressed the bodies and minds of human workers.

1973: A German company, KUKA Robotics, patented a robot featuring six axes that were electromagnetically driven.

1976: Robotics industry pioneer Victor Scheinman, a former Stanford University student who eventually became a significant figure in the robot industry and founder of Viacom Inc., sold to Unimation his patent for the Programmable Universal Manipuatlion Arm.

The Father of Artificial Intelligence

Alan Turing, a pioneer British theoretical biologist, cryptanalyst, logician, mathematician and computer scientist has been hailed as the "father of Artificial Intelligence," according to many books and articles.

Turing was instrumental in cracking the Nazi Code, leading to the end of World War II while working for the Government Code and Cypher School in Bletchley Park, the codebreaking center for the British government.

This man's many scientific discoveries were made famous by the hit 2014 Black Bear Pictures film, "The Imitation Game." Turing's inventions and discoveries helped pave the way for modern robotics, the Internet and advanced computers.

These various disciplines are collectively instrumental to various technological sectors, each vital in creating and maintaining advanced robots. These essential systems include Artificial Intelligence capable of making the devices autonomous from people.

Tragically, Turing committed suicide via cyanide poisoning in 1954 at age 41 after the British government chemically castrated him for being gay--a behavior listed as a serious crime at the time in the United Kingdom.

Turing's discoveries have been credited with likely saving hundreds of thousands or perhaps millions of lives; his codebreaking efforts enabled the Allies to end World War II in Europe earlier than otherwise would have occurred. Additionally, his various landmark discoveries leading to medical robotics have dramatically improved healthcare.

Human Genome Project Benefits

The science of robotics has benefitted significantly thanks

to the milestone Human Genome Project, where scientists mapped out each of the billions of cells and the DNA makeup of the human body.

Using this vital data since 2003, electrical engineers have been busy working in conjunction with biologists. Some of the most significant advancements stem from a resulting study of the human brain.

By understanding all simultaneous and electrical interactions within the brain during a single second, scientists are striving to build machines that mimic the seemingly magical and wonderous brain functions naturally used only by people.

Technologies that led to the Human Genone Project were made possible by various landmark discovered from the 1950s onward, significant advancements by European and American scientists. Formal planning for the project began in 1984.

Finally in 1990 in conjunction with various other countries the U.S. Congress spent several billion dollars to fund the project. The intensive research "paid off big-time" in 2003 upon the announcement that researchers had completed the effort.

Significant Discoveries Continue Rapid-Fire

Cracking the proverbial code of the human genome and DNA eventually led to the aforementioned Human Brain Project. The 10-year effort that began in 2013 has already helped pave the way for advancements in medicine, robotics and computer science.

Like electrical engineers working to advance robots, the computer experts are striving to mirror human brain function. If all goes as planned, interlinked supercomputers with massive amounts of data will instantly attempt to solve problems.

"Perhaps more than ever, various sciences and research disciplines depend on each other's discoveries," I occasionally tell physicians who inquire about this process. "None of this would have been possible without the human mind, which first envisioned these world-changing transformations."

Yet these factors also generate numerous paradoxical and

seemingly inescapable dilemmas. Everything comes down to the fact that all these advancements create living environments where people become far too dependant on technology.

"Be careful what you wish for, because you might get it," goes an age-old saying, which many of us first learn about as children. When it comes to robots, I fear, mankind has failed to do enough beforehand to envision how people will cope with these changes.

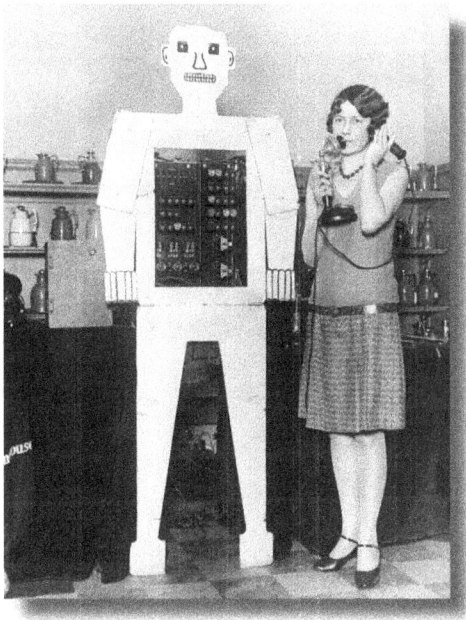

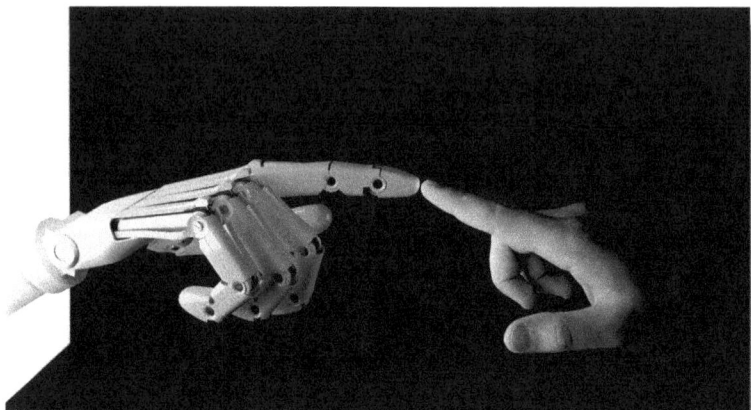

Chapter 31
Are People Too Dependent on Technology?

Any discussion or recap on the history of robotics would be remiss without delving into the serious question of whether human beings have become overly dependant on technology. The primary danger here supposedly stems from the fact that massive swaths of humanity will die if certain technologies suddenly disappear.

The advent of the Internet is often cited as a prime example. By now a huge percentage of the population realizes that if "the Web goes down," the entire infrastructure of civilized society will crash, stall, lose efficiency and become ineffective.

Virtually every major business depends on the Internet, from electric power distribution to farming, commodities trading, the stock market and transportation.

Whether society wants to hear this or not, the sad and inescapable fact remains that tens of millions of people would starve without the Internet and satellite communications. A resulting shut-down of the U.S. electrical grid would prevent the distrubition and use of gasoline essential for operating motor vehicles.

Worsening matters multi-fold, the entire healthcare industry and patients would suffer if fully dependent on robotics and digitial technology.

Beware of Becoming Overly Dependant on Medical Robots

Any shutdown or curtailment of medical robotics could cause catastrophic, wide-scale tragedies of seemingly indescribable magnitude.

Yet to this point hospital and medical clinic administrators have failed to take adequate precautions beforehand. A review of medical literature and news reports reveals little or no adequate planning in this regard.

To help put such a scenario into perspective, envision a U.S. society where every medical facility has been fully dependent on robots for more than a decade.

Then, suddenly all robot manufacturers and businesses that maintain the machines get obliterated or shut down. Even worse, the entire Internet might close due to a catastrophic event, leaving the machines without their valuable data-mining and communication processes.

When and if that happens, the medical robots would become non-functional. Worsening matters even more, any typical human physicians by that point would be incapable of performing essential medical procedures without robotic assistance. This is because most doctors by that point will lack the so-called "old-style skills" necessary to treat patients.

"Land of the Living Dead"

It is no joking matter to proclaim that the extensive and universal reliance on medical robotics would create a real-world "land of the living dead."

At some point unless adequate fail-safe systems are implemented beforehand, the average critically ill person will die without help from medical robots.

In that regard, typical hospital patients would theoretically "be dead already," because once medical and service robots shut down "the humans are doomed."

Even without advanced robots, as of 2013 the "Mother Nature Network" reported seven signs that people have become far too dependant on technology:

Work: The vast majority of people are unable to work or earn a living, if the Internet goes down for just a day--let alone for extended periods.

Lacking Human Interaction: People are increasingly having difficulty finding and communicating with "real humans," in regard to service or product delivery issues.

Loss of the Now: People are too dependant on using video and photo technology to record events, rather than actually "savoring the actual moment."

Memorization: Most people no longer memorize phone numbers, which are typically stored in their cells. Problems erupt when the phones get lost, broken or stolen.

Personal Contact: Rather than sharing one-on-one human experiences, many people are breaking up with their spouses or lovers via text messages. This robs people of the essential and growth-oriented process of actual one-on-one communication.

Brick-and-mortar stores disappear: With increased frequency actual stores that people can walk into are disappearing, replaced with Web-based delivery systems.

Cell Phone Dependence: According to numerous news reports, some people check their cell phones at least 30 times per hour--at least once every few minutes.

Medical Robotics Mimics These Flaws

As a whole, the sector of medical robotics mimics and even worsens the aforementioned flaws regarding the Internet, cell phones and computers.

Even if scientists eventually create highly functional humanoid doctors and nurses as many researchers predict, no one should ever be allowed to take away humans from healthcare.

Yes, imagine being admitted to a hospital while critically ill, during the middle of the night. The only "people" in the entire building are other bedridden patients.

Assuming that robots or people have been unable to contact your relatives, a realization hits that you might die at any moment due to severe illness or injury.

Imagine taking your dying breaths, your hand being held by a machine--rather than a real-live, pulsating, caring person.

All this certainly sounds perhaps like over-the-top science fiction. Yet such scenarios could very well play out in the near future if robotics advancements occur as planned. And, once humanity gets removed from the equation, the complete loss of any direct person-to-person interaction worldwide, what would be the use of living?

The "Spillover" Throughout Society

As if the potential healthcare industry problems are not already enough to worry about, somewhat similar issues stemming from robots are likely to permeate almost every aspect of society. Some of the greatest dangers involve the educational system.

Of course, you have already learned about the possibility that increasing numbers of colleges and universities are likely to close, according to some researchers.

Even more disturbing comes the fact that increasing numbers of instructors actually will be robots or computer-based IT systems.

Rest assured that human educators and school systems would actively fight to block or prohibit such a transition. But the sad and irreversable fact remains that robots are steadily being introduced into classroom environments worldwide.

From my view, if and when robots eventually emerge as "useful or required tools" at medical school classrooms, "the end of humanity will be closer than any of us will want to admit."

"Spooky" Transitions Have Started

Some or the "spookiest" or "freakiest" transitions in the educational system have involved telepresence robots that some school systems are introducing to classrooms.

These machines are somewhat similar to the previously mentioned devices that enable hospital patients to see images of their "living" doctors on TV screens.

According to the "Daily Mail" of London, with increased frequency students are being taught by human teachers who are actually hundreds or thousands of miles away.

In some instances, for instance, teachers located at the Nexus Academy in Columbus, Ohio, have been teaching students as far away as Arizona.

"Students said the robot felt weird at first, but it made lessons more personal," the story said. "The teacher can see the class and their work using the robot's camera."

Rapidly accelerating transitions such as these could soon make people even more dependant on robots and technology. Unless corrective measures are implemented to stop such nonsense, robots might soon become instructors in all major classrooms--including at medical schools, perhaps the world's most vital educational institutions.

Tragic Outcomes Become Possible

In just one example of such nonsense, imagine all medical schools nationwide simultaneously adopting telepresence robot instructors as a cost-saving measure.

"Such teaching would evolve into a my-way-or-the-highway infrastructure," I warn other practicing doctors who inquire about this issue. "Unless we ban such systems now early on, this technology could get installed and put into use well before we--as practicing physicians--even know what is happening."

Envision an educational environment where all students--at every medical school--simultaneously take the same exact class. In this hypothetical example, there is just one human teacher located in Boston, Massachusetts.

At a pre-appointed moment, such as 2 o'clock in the afternoon Eastern Time, the person begins instruction in basic human anatomy. Simultaneously, first-year medical students at more than 100 instituions nationwide attend this "class."

Such a system would enable medical schools to eliminate many hundreds of professorial jobs as a cost-saving measure. Equally distressing, all educational instituions would be forced to conform or adhere to just one universal view or perspective.

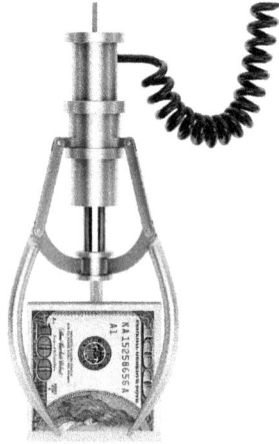

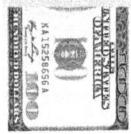

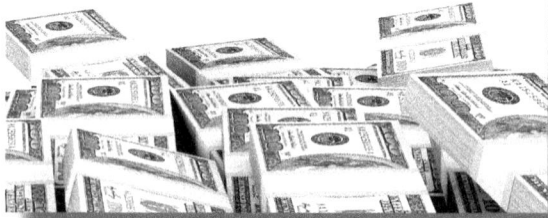

Chapter 32
Financial Questions:
Whether to Invest in Robotics Company Stocks

Using the timeless strategy of "if you can't beat them, join them," investing in robotics company stocks might serve as an advantageous strategy.

Such an investment system might become increasingly essential, as a broad spectrum of financial industry analysts insist that robots soon will replace humans in almost every job.

Of course, each person should make investment decisions only after extensive research or consulting with an financial industry professional.

Ultimately, could investing in robotics stocks lead to financial survival for people lucky enough to seize those opportunities, well before others realize what happened?

As a prime example, my researchers know of a once-successful businesswoman who wanted to invest heavily in Apple Computers when that company went public in the 1980s. But her financial planners refused to let her entertain the notion.

Subsequently, the woman's own business failed, and she has been financially struggling ever since. Sadly, today she would have a portfolio worth tens of millions of dollars if she had ignored the so-called financial experts.

Will current robotics stocks swell into the "Apples and Facebooks of the future?"

With no difinitve answers at this point, some investors are already rushing into the robotics sector--rather than risk "being left behind for good."

Who Has the Crysal Ball?

Almost everyone today over age 45 would be extremely wealthy, if having a reliable and unfailing crystal ball during their teens and 20s.

Gamblers call such an "I-should-have" perspective as proverbially "shooting rabbits," reviewing past financial results in order to visualize what "should have been, or could have been."

Such nonsense obviously can do them no good, for the so-called "time to act is now" regarding robotic stocks--well before others catch on to this already-blossoming trend.

Of course, the entire robot industry might suddenly fall flat and close. Yet that seems unlikely considering the rapid acceleration of such efforts.

"Soon, robots could be doing much more than just vacuuming your house or assembling your next car--they could also invade your investment portfolio," Chad Fraser said in a September 2015 article for "The Street" business and investment news.

Robotics Industry Business Analysis

The compelling conclusions on the robotics business as reported by "The Street" were based partly on an extensive analysis by the Boston Consulting Group.

Mirroring what electrical engineers, Internet experts and some physicians have said for many years, some financial analysts envision a financial windfall in robotics.

Like many of the aforementioned trends, these industry observers envision tremendous growth in robots for manufacturing, automation and everyday use.

"As eye-catching as these figures are, there is a good chance they may be conservative," "The Street" article said. These conclusions were revealed shortly before the International Federation of Robotics announced that during 2014 the industry's overall sales surged by a whopping 27 percent.

A simultaneous trend clicked into gear during the same period. Massive labor protests increased dramatically worldwide, as low-skilled workers joined picket lines while demanding a significant increase in the minimum wage.

Many of these people, most who lacked motivation or got poor grades when in school, started demanding wages at $15-$25 per hour.

Anti-Business Ideology Spread

The over-the-top philosophy that demands essentially "high pay" for doing mindless, repetitive work "flew in the face of common sense"--at least according to many economists and business experts.

Such concerns seemed logical. After all, who would pay for such extensive price increases? Would consumers need to do this in the form of higher prices, a process that could criple an already tenuous or weakened economy?

Or, perhaps even worse, would almost all businesses in general have to accept significanlty lower profit margins or even possible bankruptcy due to an over-the-top, government-mandated increase in the minimum wage?

From the view of at least some investors and business operators, the logical solution would be to use robots to eliminate the jobs of uneducated people who demand significantly higher wages--merely for doing "mindless and repetitive" work.

As a prime example, consider typical fast-food restaurant burger flippers during the late 2010s. Rather than boost their wages to exorbitant levels that would cripple the industry, such businesses could replace the workers with efficient robots.

Businesses Seize Advantages

Whether business executives like to admit this or not, the Rise of the Robots is coming at a potentially ideal time for economy--at least in this regard.

Everything comes down to the fact that over-the-top regulations and liberal governments have been making it impossible for most businesses to function--let alone succeed at any efforts to generate huge profits.

With these factors in mind, business analysts realize that the vast majority of today's most prosperous and successful businesses are technology-based. For the most part these are Web-oriented companies that lack any need for tens of thousands of employees. The prime examples are Facebook, Alphabet and Amazon.

Yet these instances mark only the beginning of the surging automation trend, since the vast majority of companies still need massive numbers of robots. Once this change occurs, many people will no longer be picketing for higher wages--primarily because jobs will become non-existent for low-educated people.

"Watch carefully, because seemingly within the blink of an eye, these transitions will occur," I tell some medical industry observers. "Also, just as they have depended on reliable employees until now, most business sectors--including hospitals and medical clinics--will become increasingly dependant on robots."

On the negative side, almost any business that fails or refuses to "recruit robots" into its overall operations likely will become doomed to failure and eventual closure.

The Many Positives for Business

As the general public and most business sectors become increasingly interested in robots, the many potential benefits for companies are becoming undeniable. Among some of the most critical factors:

Health Insurance: Without human employees, businesses no longer get saddled with ludicrous requirements that the companies pay for health insurance--as mandated by Obamacare. Eliminating such costs would increase profit, while boosting efficiency.

Buying Robots: Mirroring trends from most emerging technologies, the per-unit costs of buying robots is likely to decrease as such devices saturate the economy. In a sense, this is like digital TVs that initially cost thousands of dollars, before prices decreased sharply to hundreds of dollars. Similar cost reductions occurred in the personal computer and smartphone industries.

Improved Efficiency: In general, robots are designed to sharply increase efficiency, while eliminating any need to "coddle or babysit" whiny, complaining and non-productive people. For many businesses--including the healthcare sector--having only a handful of employees, instead of hundreds or thousands, likely would be far easier to manage. Productivity might increase substantially as a result.

Human Resources: Companies that successfully or seamlessly replace most or all employees might be able to downsize or eliminate expensive human resources departments. This could sharply boost profitability. Some businesses would no longer need to continually find and replace certain highly qualified employees.

Medical Industry Benefits: Some of the biggest potential cost savings would benefit the healthcare industry, as certain high-paid nurses and staff-level personnel have their jobs eliminated by robots. Thus, investing in publicly traded hospital stocks might emerge as a hugely profitable strategy for some investors, particularly the shares of institutions that are becoming fully digitalized.

Misinformation Confuses the Public

Worsening problems multi-fold, college professors and people fashioning themselves as robotics experts started giving the public conflicting details on how these machines will impact society, the economy and the job market. Some of these so-called "gurus" have even given conflicting information on which jobs will be endangered.

A prime example of such reckless and irresponsible statements occurred on January 17, 2016, when Silicon Valley businessman Martin Ford discussed these issues on a popular radio program hosted by investment expert Bob Brinker. Ford discussed details from his book, "Rise of the Robots: Technology and the Threat of a Jobless Future"--a "New York Times" bestseller released in May 2015 by Basic Books.

According to various published reports, during the final one-hour segment of Brinker's three-hour program, Ford made numerous misstatements regarding the impact that robotics will have on the job market.

One of Ford's most blatant oversights on Brinker's program occurred when he proclaimed that people with blue collar jobs are most likely to have machines impact their professions. This assertion was contrary to what streams of certified economics and robotics experts who have said--that everyone from accountants, lawyers and doctors will eventually have their professions adversely impacted or even decimated by machines.

Statements such as Ford's should motivate business professionals, consumers and current or prospective university students to remain wary of such recommendations or commentary from so-called "robotics professionals."

Indeed, relying on a single news report or just one robotics book when making a life-changing decision might put a person on a negative, irreversable and potentially destructive course in life. Adding to the confusion, during the radio interview Ford either blatantly overlooked or just plain failed to acknowledge the countless advancements in robotics during the eight-month span from his book's release until he appeared on Brinker's show.

Non-Stop Developments Surge in Robotics

My non-scientific, informal review indicates that from around 10 to 30 unique new stories on extensive robotics developments get released daily. These articles appear in everything from massive online news sources such as MSN.com to the "New York Times," "USA Today," and small community newspapers.

Some of the biggest disparities and inconsistencies come in the form of online videos on YouTube or blog postings that often give sharply different predictions on how society can or should cope with--or prepare for--the international and regional economic impacts that robots will cause in the coming decades.

According to a popular blog on "blogspot" called "Honey's Bob Brinker Beehive Buzz," on the January 2016 program, the widely acclaimed financial expert and radio host questioned Ford's hint that people who lose their jobs to robots will still have a "guaranteed income."

To his great credit, Brinker--almost always heralded as a sound-minded and well-reasoned expert in personal and business finances--questioned Ford's contention that the funds going to such unemployed people will come from "taxes of some sort."

Using his well-informed but gentle "in-your-face" style, Brinker then pointed out to Ford that California's combined federal, state and local tax rate was already 57 percent--a total that many people content makes living or doing business in the Golden State impossible.

Then, Ford responded by saying that people do not lose their incentive to work until taxes reach 60 percent to 70 percent.

"Ford then helpfully reminded Bob and listeners that the marginal tax rate does not apply to all dollars a person earns--'just the last dollar,'" the blog said. "Bob then straightened him out on this, telling him the marginal tax rate applies to all dollars earned above a certain amount. *Thank you Bob*."

So-Called Experts Sometimes Spread Incorrect Details

Either ignorant of the truth or ignoring streams of robotics developments since his book's release, during the same program Ford also gave additional commentary on the Rise of the Robots--some helpful, while other observations seemed misleading. Among Ford's comments, plus my analysis on the accuracy of his statements:

Workplace changes: Ford contends that generally machines are encroaching on human capabilities at work, a blanket or "coverall" statement that just about all experts agree with.

Repetitive work: He urged people to avoid getting "repetitive work," which many officials agree will be the first type of jobs that robots will replace or fill on a massive scale.

Self-Improvement: In perhaps one of his most ill-informed comments, Ford urged listeners of Brinker's show to impove their skills while expanding their creativity. Yet in saying this, Ford ignored the fact that significant advancements in Artificial Intelligence already were well underway--at the same time as scientists started creating, designing and building machines with "skills" equal to--or even far more superior than--today's humans in the general economic marketplace.

Worker Categories: Right on the mark, Ford said that robotics advancements likely will make both blue collar and white collar workers vulnerable to changes in their work environment or even job losses. Yet either misinformed or lacking enough detail, Ford said that medical professionals who rarely or never interact personally with patients are the only such workers who will be impacted by robotics. To the contrary, however, he failed to mention long-term AI developments that many experts insist will impact those professions within several decades--even professionals who now interact with patients.

Creativity: In perhaps his most damaging oversight, Ford urged college students to pursue creative career choices. Sadly, Brinker's listeners were never told that robots, automated programs and digital-based systems are increasingly being used as actors, writers, artists, photographers, and even "creativity consultants." As a result, many people who follow Ford's advice in this regard might soon find themselves among the jobless individuals that he insists that government will protect with an assured income.

More Urgent Reasons for Concern Emerged

In perhaps one of his most lame and misguided comments on Brinker's program, Ford also mentioned what he described as the fact that--from the end of World War II to the 1970s--wages increased thanks to improvements in machines.

Ford "seemed to be saying that workers reaped the

financial rewards for the increased productivity that was due to machines," the Honey blog said. "Wages have stagnated since then for all except those at the top of the income distribution.

"Bob asked whether workers should get 'real' wage increases--not just due to inflation--'for just showing up.'" According to the blog, Ford answered: "That is the way it has been; it has become an expectation."

But Brinker kept pushing the issue, asking, "How much is up to the worker ... To earn real wage increases?"

Ford answered that workers must increase their skills, while the government has a responsibility to provide the necessary education--but that doing so might not be sufficient. Understandably, according to the blog, this lead to comments about guaranteed incomes and about how people should start thinking about changing societal rules.

From my view, such assumptions are "pure speculation," since changing the standard work-for-pay system will decimate business and ultimately the entire economy. Such a process would either verge on--or even become--socialism, which has already proven itself as a failure in numerous countries that have tried socialism.

Robotics Stocks

As with almost every other significant stock investment, robotics company stock prices are likely to be cyclical, moving up and down over time, analysts say.

This means some companies are likely to be "hot" or "popular" for periods, while other firms are at least temporarily "tepid"--a percentage of them eventually surging in price.

By late 2015, some of the most frequently mentioned "hot stocks" in the robotics sector were:

Alphabet-Google: Many investors might have failed to realize this at the time, but this company's shares had surged during the previous six months--largely because of its acquisitions of potentially profitable robotics firms. Investors were lured by contracts that some of these various sub-companies had with the U.S. Army, Navy and Marines. At the time, Google's online advertising services amassed 90 percent of Alphabet's revenues. So, targeting its robotics divisions for revenue growth were considered part of a "solidified" long-term investment strategy. Some investors viewed this as a good method, especially as military robot development surged while the battle against terrorism intensified.

Yaskawa Electronics: Traded under the symbol YASKY, this Japanese-based firm held an estimated 20 percent of the industrial robotics market. Yaskawa's corporate forecasts expected company revenues to triple by 2025. While the company's robots performed on factory floors worldwide, according to published reports at least one analysts called this stock "the best robot play."

ABB Limited: Traded under the symbol ABB, this Switzerland-based firm with a $43 billion market cap specializes in robotics that work on circuit breakers, switch gear, transformers and the infrastructure of power grids. Some analysts theorized that the company would eventually spin off its fast-growing automation business, breaking from its slow-growth utility sector.

iRobot: Traded under the symbol IRBT, this company's many popular machines include an automated lawnmower that remained in the development stage. Although the company had a market cap of only $885 million--relatively small in the investment world--"Morningstar" reported that its Roomba robotic vacuum sales increased 18 percent within the home market. Besides producing robots for the U.S. military, the company also manufactured automated cleaners of floors, pools and gutters. Sales increased 24 percent during a single quarter of 2014, thanks to increased revenues from China and growth in the company's security and defense businesses.

Ekso Bionics Holdings: This previously mentioned Richmond, California-based firm specializing in healthcare robotics is traded under the symbol EKSO. Some financial analysts consider its exoskeleton rehab devices as well positioned in a sector with tremendous growth, potentially serving up to 2.5 million Americans with disabilities. The potential goes to other industries as well, thanks to Esko products that can sharply boost the strength of people wearing them--such as military personnel. At the time, though, investment analysts categorized Esko as a thinly traded over-the-counter stock--with a market cap of merely $139 million. Even so, at least from the view of some investment advisors Esko was an early-stage tech company with huge potential.

Upside Potential: Medical Robotics Stocks

Within the overall robotics sector, numerous companies outside home services and industrial applications included firms making machines specializing in health care.

Many of these companies had not yet reached big-name status, partly because the firms specialized within a specific industry. Even so, at least from the view of some investment advisors, several of these companies were worthy of consideration as potentially lucrative investments. Among those occasionally mentioned in news reports:

Intuitive Surgical Inc.: Traded under the symbol ISRG, this company provides robot-assisted surgical devices to more than 2,000 hospitals worldwide. Its products include the previously mentioned da Vinci Surgical Systems.

Mazor Robotics Ltd.: Traded under the symbol MZOR, the company produces robots that assist in tens of thousands of spine surgeries worldwide. One of the firm's most significant developments occurred in 2013, when its Renaissance Guidance System was used in the world's first successful lumbar spine fusion surgery.

Hansen Medical, Inc.: Traded under the symbol HNSN, this California-based firm briefly mentioned earlier, has many robotics medical applications. These range from catheters to intra-vascular procedures.

Accuray Incorporated: Traded under the symbol ARAY,

this Sunnyvale, California-based firm designs, develops and sells radiosurgery and radiation therapy systems for treating tumors. Its most widely known products include the CyberKnife System used in stereotatic surgery. The CyberKnife treatment protocol strives to minimize damage to non-diseased areas of the body. The company's TomoTherapy H Series product breaks radiation beams into a collection of smaller beams; this process enables physicians to precisely target specific tumors with greater accuracy.

Bright Long-Term Outlook

A review of analysts' comments on medical robotics stocks showed little negative commentary, but rather an overall positive outlook from analysts.

"Now that the heat is on to make healthcare more affordable and to ensure better outcomes, robotics are getting a new lease on life in the medical community," said an "Investor Place" report on the industry. This is a "shot in the arm that could make the right companies the high-growth healthcare stocks of the future."

In fact, according to a report from "Transparency Market Research," the global medical robotics systems market was expected to grow from $5.48 billion in 2011 to $13.6 billion in 2018--well before the advent of even more advanced technology.

"Although medical robots are likely to experience the most significant growth in revenue, other systems in fields such as non-invasive radiosurgery, prosthetics and exoskeletons, and assistive and rehabilitation robots also smell strongly of opportunity," the "Investor Place" article said. "Not surprisingly, the key drivers of medical robotics are the same game-changing factors impacting healthcare stocks: industry automation; a greying population with motion-restricting conditions; and advances in non-invasive surgical procedures."

Partly for these reasons, the story suggested considering investments in Intuitive Surgical, iRobot and Ekso.

Chapter 33

Robotics Clubs Rapidly Spread Worldwide

Latching on to the fast-growing robotics field, students at most major colleges and universities worldwide have launched robotics clubs in recent years.

This has emerged from a "mere trend" into a highly acceptable process, so groundbreaking and essential that high schools worldwide have launched similar clubs.

Any family that wants their children and young adults to have potentially lucrative jobs in the future should make joining these organizations "a must."

In fact, these efforts are considered so essential that I personally have developed numerous recommendations. Among them:

Parents: To help ensure that your child or young-adult offspring gets positioned for a job, encourage them to join and actively participate in such organizations.

Jobs: Participating in such clubs might position participants to "become stronger job candidates" upon reaching full-time working age.

Tools: Families that can afford to should consider purchasing robot-production kits for their teens and young-adult relatives.

Studies: Besides joining and participating in such clubs, these young people should concentrate on the various previously mentioned subjects--topics likely to increase their chances of eventually landing robotics industry employment.

Personal Connections: Besides merely participating in clubs and those organizations' related contests, the members should actively establish connections with adult instructors or representatives of robotics companies who attend competitions.

Focus on Success

Focusing on these aforementioned strategies could play a signicant role in determing your young family member's long-term economic survival.

Remember, as stated in early chapters, our incompetent government and politicians have done nothing to plan for society's financial survival amid robots.

At least for now, until any positive government policy changes on this matter, young people and their families are responsible for making their own decisions on this.

"The time to take positive action is right now without delay, rather than waiting," I sometimes say. "You owe yourself and your family these essential basics. To do otherwise would be to court potential financial disaster for all of your younger relatives."

Yes, very soon the days will be gone forever where people make their lifelong plans during childhood with only "human interaction" as the most critical factor. From this point forward, you and your relatives must factor "robots into your life-long plan."

Finding Appropriate Clubs

Right off the bat, parents and even grandparents have an urgent responsibility to encourage and to help give their young offspring guidance in this regard.

A critical and necessary first step involves locating an acceptable and safe local robotics club for your young relatives to consider. Just as important, because "it's never too late to learn," adults also can join at least some of these organizations.

Among the basic ways to locate such a club:

Internet search: Use your favorite search engine such as Google to type in "robotics club" followed by the name of your community. This invariably will generate a list of local options, including organizations and participants.

School inquiries: Check with the office of your child's

school. Many elementary schools, middle schools, high schools and almost every university has such programs. If the school does not have such a club, in all likelihood it probably can recommend one.

Teachers and classmates: Especially as interest in robotics increases, lots of teachers and plenty of your child's classmates will know of the "hottest, most popular" robotics clubs or machine-oriented programs.

Participation Requirements and Fees
Many robotics clubs are free to join or have minimal entry fees. Particularly if cost is a major factor for your family, be sure to ask beforehand about required expenses.

Assistance: Low-income families should ask if financial assistance is available for club membership, or if "free" participation is allowed for those in such circumstances.

Recommendations: Ask lots of teachers and participants for their advice on costs, particularly suggestions from those who have been involved for awhile.

Safety: Be sure to ask about safety issues, such as dangers from machines--plus whether video monitoring is done to ensure your child is safe from potentially dangerous people.

Time considerations: Check to determine if the club's meeting times coincide with your child's study and play schedules.

Cooperation: Try to find a club where your child will be encouraged to cooperate and interact intellectually with other students and teachers.

Make the Process Fun
Strive to encourage the club to have fun-filled activities, in part because huge percentages of today's youngsters have relativley low attention spans.

"If it isn't fun, don't do it," some people might say. "For some of us, activities are not worth doing unless they are exciting and exhilerating to the mind and body."

Largely for these reasons, most robotics clubs for middle school, high school and even university students have regularly scheduled competitions.

This serves as an ingenious learning strategy, since the vast majority of human beings are somewhat competitive by nature--at least to varying degrees.

A continual desire to "win" serves as a primary reason many robotics clubs strive to invent or create new applications for the machines. Some of the clubs' most popular competitions involves robots built to battle each other in a "miniaturized arena" setting, such as a screened-off area atop a basketball court.

Necessary Equipment Requirements

Some schools or clubs provide the necessary equipment, while others encourage members to purchase their own materials for producing, managing or maintaining the machines. The basic equipment can involve:

Robot kits: These toolsets or parts usually contain all the materials necessary to build a basic, rudimentary or crude version of specific types of robots.

Purchase venues: Many kits can be purchased online from major sellers or distributors such as Amazon.com. Department stores also sometimes offer the kits.

Kit costs: Expenses usually depend on the specific model of robot, with per-kit fees ranging from less than $100, to hundreds or even thousands of dollars.

Maintenance: Check your current or prospective club's rules to determine who is responsible for storing and maintaining your youngster's robotics kit or tools.

Give "Good Reasons"

For a variety of reasons including shyness or low self-esteem, some teens or young adults might balk at the very notion of joining or participating in robotics clubs.

Parents, grandparents or legal guardians who encounter this obstacle can consider taking a positive approach when striving to encourage such activities.

Online learning applications and kits designed for home use often are among the most frequently mentioned options in such circumstances.

In recent decades psychologists have encouraged adults to "actively listen" to their youngsters, partly to understand the person's desires, fears or motivations. Largely in an effort to avoid pushing the child, teen or young adult away emotionally, parents should refrain from being judgmental, nagging or being "holier-than-thou."

All along, casually mention that having such basic or advanced skills can help make the young person employable or even a viable candidate for a high-paying robotics industry job.

Refrain from getting discouraged if the young person balks or scoffs at such suggestions, even in instances where they complain to you that "these clubs don't make sense," or even "I don't care about it."

With equal emphasis, you also might mention that learning the details of robots serves as an essential way to maintain, operate or control domestic machines. Keep in mind that domestic robots are slated to enter household environments at an accelerated pace throughout the 2020s.

Club Popularity Surges

High school robot clubs were surging in popularity worldwide and particularly within the United States and Japan, at least judging by a steady steam of news reports.

Particularly as reported by small newspapers in local markets, mainstream media stories often feature images of cheering teenagers at robotics competitions.

The excitement has catapulted into many universities as well, with top teams intensifying competition at the collegiate level.

Human members of robotics teams placing high or emerging victorious sometimes position themselves for potentially lucrative job offers from burgeoning robotics companies or even establsihed firms.

Yet challenges have emerged for some programs, particularly at the high school level, at least according to some news stories.

Robotics Club Growth Challenges Teachers

Some teachers in Southern California were beginning to "grumble" about working conditions as high-tech robotics programs skyrocket in popularity, according to a 2015 article in the "San Diego Union Tribune."

"They cite long-simmering disputes with school district administrators who they say won't pay them the same stipends as football or basketball coaches, band directors or advisors to other programs," the story said.

The issue became so heated in Soutern California that some robotics instructors began demanding more compensation, according to the article. Like instructors in sports and music programs, the robotics pros spend additional time aside from their regular work hours.

Amid such complaints, school district administrators nationwide apparently have found themselves essentially stuck in a quandry. These officials are being forced into a proverbial balancing act.

Besides striving to maintain a "fair" system for all programs, public school district administrators need to comply with various federal and state funding requirements. The issue seems to be heating up on a broad scale as school districts and universities face increasingly tight budgets.

Make Robotics a High Priority

Rather than striving to essentially "sweep this issue under the rug," public school and university administrators need to address the issue head-on.

The basic and essential question comes down to whether economic survival via robots is more important to society than football games.

As disturbing as this question might seem, "is it more essential for society to produce men and women who excel at sports, or should priorities focus on high-tech machines that will profoundly impact all of our lives in the near future?"

Also, rather than relegating all robotics instructions to "just the clubs," should high schools and universities launch required basic instruction on the building, maintenance and use of such machines?

Quite disturbingly, the vast majority of university and school district board members seem to lack the basic understanding of how important robotics is becoming to society. To ignore this issue, while blatantly refusing to launch robotics classes and funded clubs, our educational systems are creating a profound disservice to society.

Acknowledge Society's Heroes

People everywhere should consider today's low-paid or non-paid university and public school robotics club instructors as "today's unsung heroes helping all of society."

Some receive only several hundred dollars monthly, or less than $3,000 yearly, for all this additional effort.

Sadly, because these duties are handled on top of their regular teaching hours, these adults have less time to enjoy or enhance their personal lives.

So, rather than merely raising their stipends, these essential teachers and adult robotics club managers also should get well-deserved public recognition.

Of course, no one can mandate how the local media should report on these efforts. Yet with encouragement from parents and even club members, perhaps regional newspapers and TV stations can give robotics competitions as much coverage as high school or college football games.

Another Issue: Space for Clubs

As if the pay issue were not already enough to worry about, a huge percentage of robotics club instructors face the additional problem of finding adequate meeting and work space for their teams.

The vast majority of school buildings lack adequate space dedicated to building, storing or maintaining robots, particularly at the middle and high school level.

Club instructors often spend significant time striving to get space for the clubs.

Added to this comes the disturbing fact that booster or alumni organizations already push the bulk of their political power and funds toward sports programs.

As a result, I sometimes proclaim, "the system is already set up to keep robotics at the bottom of the proverbial totem pole. In doing so, we're sending a negative message to young people-- regarding the priorities that today's society should have."

Move Forward in a Positive Manner

On the positive side, many school robotics clubs are moving foward in a positive manner. This is so vital that some clubs might actually help to pave the way for technological advancements that robotics companies lack time or resources to achieve.

Among the many positive factors made possible by these groups:

Creativity: Instructors at many clubs encourage students to get creative; this helps activate both regions of the pupils' minds--the visionary and analytical realms.

Teamwork: Like most sports, the best and most effective robotics teams sometimes emerge as successful when participants work together as a cohesive unit; for the clubs, primary tasks include building machines or creating revolutionary concepts.

Friendships: Like school sports participants, robotics club members can develop strong friendships or life-long emotional bonds with teammates.

Positive activities: Remember that age-old saying, "Idleness is the devil's workshop." Well, although in-depth studies apparently have never been done on this, chances seem strong that remaining super-busy with robotics club activities might "rob students of time" that they might otherwise use getting into trouble.

Additional Positives Emerged

While some school districts nationwide lag far behind in efforts to boost robotics instruction, to their great credit numerous regions have excelled in this regard.

Among the positive, prime examples here is in Goshen, Indiana, where public school students get robotics instruction in daytime classrooms from the third grade through high school--plus opportunities to participate in after-school robot clubs.

This is a particularly remarkable and noteworthy achievement by school administrators, especially when considering the fact that just a few years before launching the program, the schools' robotics activities were relegated to summer camp, according to the "Goshen News."

In an article by Julie Crothers Beer, the newspaper described this as an "exciting time" for the Wawasee Community Schools Corporation. The robotics instruction is part of the schools' efforts to focus on STEM--science, technology, engineering and math.

The article quoted Kim Nguyen, the Wawasee Area Career and Technical Cooperative's director, as saying that the Project Lead the Way Engineering and Biomedical Science and computer coding classes had been offered at the high school level for a number of years.

"What we wanted to do was create a pathway from elementary to high school to start preparing students with a better set of skills in these areas to graduate from our high school--and hopefully to move into these careers in their future," Nguyen told the newspaper.

Fourth and fifth graders receive about two weeks of instructions that feature compelling demonstrations, such as teaching robots how to roll on the floor in pre-designated patterns. At that earlier age, said one teacher, this is "just enough to peak their interest and hopefully infect them with the robotics bug."

Significant Advancements

By late 2015, streams of news stories were being issued almost daily about the positive developments of high school and college robotics clubs

These clubs collectively and indivdually already seemed to be playing a significant role in the enhancement of robots, expanding the machines' capabilities.

Amazingly, however, the general public seemed oblivious to these changes, which eventually could have profound impacts on healthcare and many other industries.

Average families nationwide could not be blamed for remaining ignorant on this issue, because the mainstream media generally ignored these groundbreaking stories.

"Every significant journey in life begins with a first step," an age-old saying tells us. "The most important phase in reaching any destination is to simply begin the journey."

Well, as society begins the seemingly unstoppable transition into robotics, the same holds true for families and young people. To purposely ignore these developments would be to deny yourself and your family of essential knowledge.

Praise Those Courageous Enough to Persevere

At all times we should remember an additional long-time saying, keen words of wisdom at this time: "If you cannot beat them, join them."

This especially holds true for anyone adamant against the Rise of the Robots, because the significant changes are well underway--whether we want that or not.

Among just some of the many countless advencements already being developed by robotics clubs, as reported by various news stories:

Trash Disposal: Public school students in Dickson County, Iowa, were developing robots to automatically collect and sort trash, according to a story in the "Dickson County News." Teams used Legos-brand toys as essential parts of their robot designs, competing against other participants in developing the most efficient machines.

After School Clubs: Students were encouraged to join an after-school robotics club at a Boys and Girls Club in Starr County, Texas, according to that community's "The Monitor" newspaper. These clubs are affiliated with the aforementioned popular program, STEM--blending science, technology, engineering and math. Participants have many STEM-affiliated clubs that they can join, each focused on studies that range from computer technology to oceanography.

Battling Robots: Students at Saint Mary's Catholic Secondary School in Hamilton, a community in Ontario, Canada, were among competitors who engage in built-from-scratch robot battles, according to "The Hamilton County Spectator." Independent of that article, robotics experts say such efforts might emerge as significant in improving the rapidly growing sector of military robots.

Playing Catch-Up: Some public school districts without robotics teams were struggling to catch up with other regions that already had basic, mid-level or advanced clubs. At Smithfield-Selma Senior High School in Johnson County, North Carolina, school officials organized its 15th Annual Digital Technology Expo--but waited until 2015 to launch its first robotics club for students.

Student Independence: At Belton High School and Belton New Tech High School in Texas, students in the schools' robotics clubs are encouraged or allowed to make independent decisions on their creations--autonomous from their adult teachers. Students from higher grade levels help mentor the younger participants, according to the "TDT News." The club's main focus is the annual BEST competition, which stands for Boosting Engineering, Science and Technology.

University Robot Teams

Robot teams at universities nationwide had already accelerated to sophisticated levels, attracting help and cooperation from many major institutions.

The specific level of how much medical schools might be cooperating in this overall process seemed relatively unclear. Yet judging from various news reports the advancements made by these efforts seemed significant on a broad scale.

The college-level efforts got at least some nationwide news coverage, while high school-level clubs remained relatively ignored--even by local media outlets. Among some of the most significant university robotics team advancements:

NASA: The U.S. government's famed National Aeronautics and Space Administration became so impressed with advancements in college-level robotics teams, that the agency selected two universities to assist in a milestone effort. According to NBC News, NASA selected the Massachusetts Institute of Technology and Northeastern University to help upgrade and design advancements for the agency's R5 humanoid robot--which someday might help explore deep space or even Mars. The story also said that NASA envisioned that the R5 could "someday be used in space missions, either performing tasks before humans arrive or working alongside the human crew."

Club Growth: Like the high school-level clubs, which have far more teams in some communities or states than others, the number of such organizations at the university level seemed somewhat sporadic--at least on a nationwide basis. For instance, the "Daily Courier" in Prescott, Arizona, reported that there were "only" eight or nine university-level robotics teams in The Grand Canyon State. "VEX Robotics Design System primarily serves as a platform for students from elementary school up to university levels, to learn about, build and compete with robots," said the "Courier" article by Max Efrein. "The organization operates on an international scale and organizes U.S. state competitions, as well as a world competition that is often held in the U.S."

Significant Advancements: Robotics clubs and structured learning programs focused on such machines remained busy creating a wide variety of advancements. Brilliant students at Western University in London, Ontario, Canada, participated in a program where each pupil monitors separate aspects of NASA's Opportunity and Curiosity robots on Mars. According to a news story by the "Weather Network," the students' assignments cover everything from management, science and mapping to monitoring cameras and scientific instruments.

Club Improvements Needed

University and public school administrators need to do much more to improve robotics clubs, particularly within the healthcare sector.

At least judging by news reports, the infrastructure of today's medical schools seems to lack in-depth and cohesive integration with robotics advancements.

A tragic danger becomes possible if this apparent oversight is allowed to continue. The key factors here remain impossible to ignore. Among them:

Communication: Starting now rather than later, medical school professors, current doctors and perhaps advanced students need to play a role in developing robotics communication and software systems.

Open Forums: Medical schools, in conjunction with robotic teams and companies building the devices, need to organize, host and publicize more open public forums. Everyone needs an opportunity to openly discuss these critical issues, especially without fear of any potential reprisal if mentioning topics that some people consider insensitive.

Funding Issues: Authorities need to clearly address

funding for such efforts, particularly amid the continual budget-tightening process that continues unabated at most institutions of higher education.

In summary, the many various robotics clubs and university-level classes on this topic might steadily play an essential role in improving medical treatment. Yet if left unchecked or unregulated, a danger will remain that only a finite number of robotics and pharmaceutical companies will get an "inside track" in dominating the healthcare industry. Such an outcome could generate monopolies, while sharply increasing medical costs and potentially forcing doctors, hospitals and diagnosticians to rely solely on certain robot brands or models.

Just as essential, as briefly mentioned much earlier, medical experts and associations need to get much more involved in setting the treatment protocol instilled within healthcare robots. These officials also need to regulate or identify the informational databases that medical robots use to retrieve information.

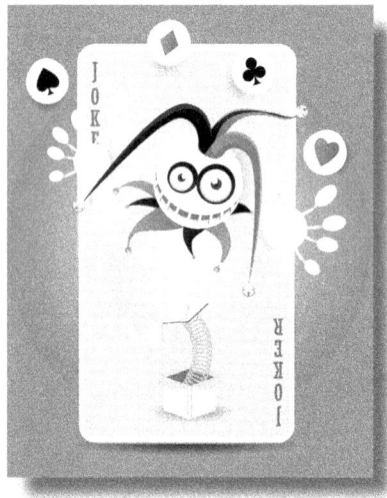

Chapter 34
Military and Police Robots

Advanced robots under continual development for the military and police likely will have a profound impact on medicine and the healthcare industry as a whole.

The rush to develop deadly and difficult-to-destroy military machines intensified, to the point where some analysts recalled the Great Space Race of the 1960s.

Streams of news reports well into the 2010s described intense efforts by the United States, Russia and China to build the most powerful and deadly robotic soldiers.

The publicity became so intense that some anti-killer robot organizations protested, demanding that politicians worldwide ban the creation and production of such machines.

Fears centered on the likelihood that such devices likely would be able to conquor entire countries and cities at a rapid-fire rate.

Critics claimed that under worst-case scenarios military robots would be able to knock down buildings, withstand firefights without sustaining damage, and quickly crush all humans within entire regions.

Medical Applications Necessary

The steady development of military robots increased speculation that authorities would also need to accelerate healthcare capabilities to treat victims of this technology.

Like the American Civil War of the 1860s, the robot armies likely will increase the widespread need for quick and considerable advancements in medicine.

Through that pivotal phase in human history more than 150 years ago, doctors rushed to develop or increase the use of relatively new painkillers for soldiers severely wounded in battle.

At the time, ball-shaped bullets ripped apart limbs and

torsos of many thousands of warriors, generating carnage never experienced before on such an instantaneous and massive scale.

Wounds suffered by people encountering military robots likely will generate a new type of wound, primarily laser burns and the crushing of limbs. In all probability, many thousands or even millions of people simultaneously will suffer similar wounds--if and when such a widespread battle erupts.

Disturbing Media Reports
According to a maze of disturbing media stories, typical humans could find themselves incapable of defending themselves against super-powerful military robots.

The race to develop advanced versions of these machines was expected to triple from 2013 to 2019, reaching $12 billion, according to a November 2015 article in "Run Direct Magazine."

These efforts began largely in an attempt to devise ways to protect U.S. soldiers from improvised explosive devices, a problem that intensified during the Iraq and Afghanistan wars.

"The wider market for military ground robots will develop as a mechanism to fight terrorism in response to the bombings in Boston and elsewhere," the story said. "Bombings of civilians is a very serious matter and needs to be addressed with mobile platforms that prevent terrorist acts."

If efforts continue as planned by the U.S. government, by 2020 or perhaps even much sooner the military robots will be able to destroy entire human armies or even cultures.

These Dangers Impact Healthcare
Many of these advanced and seemingly unstoppable weapons will have a potentially negative impact on healthcare--primarily within countries targeted by warring military robots.

Assuming that robotics advancements occur as planned, all human doctors within entire regions could be quickly killed or severely injured by the machines during such a war.

In all likelihood, widespread devastation would continue

non-stop until military leaders "order" the robots to stop killing, or the machines' programming tells them to "cease fire."

Specific details have not yet been revealed on how officials expect or want healthcare providers to adapt to these horrific challenges.

Yet chances seem strong or even likely that authorities already were well along in the process of developing quick emergency medical responses to such attacks. To do otherwise, ignoring the situation, would essentially doom all people within any society or nation threatened by advanced, powerful and heavily armed military robots.

More "Real" Than a 1950s B-Movie

From the view of many people, the mere notion of such warfare seems about as plausible as a cheap, low-grade 1950s science fiction movie.

Yet streams of news reports from reliable or credible news services and publications in recent years have said otherwise--that the situation is indeed "real."

The "WhaTech" report on technological advancements revealed in November 2015 that the surge in military robots continued unabated.

"The military charter is shifting to provide protection against terrorists and people seek to maintain a safe, mobile, independent lifestyle," the story said. "Much of the military mission is moving to adopt a police force training mission, seeking to achieve protection of civilian populations on a worldwide basis."

According to a study mentioned by the article, the rate of advancements in military robots will hinge primarily on how much funding governments allocate for the efforts.

World Domination Becomes Possible

The country or countries emerging as the first to develop highly destructive miltiary robots--produced and used on a massive scale--is likely to dominate international politics and culture, at least according to numerous news reports.

Among the first prototypes was "Spot," an electronic dog developed to engage in warfare along with human military personnel, according to a November 2015 story in the "Christian Science Monitor."

In conjunction with the previously mentioned Alphabet-Google company, Boston Dynamics, the U.S. Marine Corps assisted the "training" or programming of these machines. Soldiers and engineers tested the devices in the hills, urban areas and woodland of Virginia.

This specific effort was just one of many military robotics development programs continuing on a non-stop basis worldwide--particularly in the U.S., China and Russia.

Without exaggeration, although the general public learned little or nothing about these developments, the situation emerged into the modern-day equivalent of the notorious nuclear arms race--which peaked from the 1950s through 1970s.

Envision Potential Outcomes

Unlike nuclear bomb attacks that would destroy, flatten, and radiate entire cultures, high-functioning military robots could kill or wound everyone--in some instances without causing significant property damage.

In order to maximize casualties, the machines likely would attack all human personnel in hospitals. Devilish people controlling these robots might program the devices to "spare" as much of the healthcare infrastructre as possible; that way the same facilities could eventually be used by people who own or control the machines.

Ideally, at least from the view of scientists and engineers developing military robots, countries with these machines would be able to pulverize any nation, culture or social that lacks such robots.

Besides lasers and bombs, physically pulverizing or even

capturing adversaries might be an option. Among the most likely human targets marked for capture or death probably would be human doctors, nurses and anyone with healthcare expertise.

While under continual attack or threats from Palestinians and other Middle Eastern adversaries, the nation of Israel had a unique "RoboTeam" operating in the U.S.--working to devise military robots, according to the "Globes" online news service.

Initially Used as Assistants

During the earliest stages of development, military robots will be developed and used to assist human military personnel.

The "Globes" article quoted Yosi Wolf, the RoboTeam's co-CEO, as saying that many large companies are making military robots--for use in every country where the U.S. military operates.

"When you say 'RoboCop,' people usually think about a robot replacing a soldier, but that's not right," Wolf told "Globes." "A robot is an effective work tool that facilitates better work."

Yet contrary to the perspectives of Wolf and some engineers, critics of the process including internationally acclaimed physicist Stephen Hawking contend otherwise; they claim that "autonomous or independently functioning" devices would be the next step in the ongoing development and rollout of military robots.

Remember that as previously mentioned, rather than continually being operated or controlled by people, autonomous robots are programmed to "make decisions" on their own. This "choosing process" would be controlled or mandated by a mixture of AI technologies, coupled with movements or actions that the devices have been pre-programmed to make.

Delving into the realm of seemingly unbelievable sci-fi, at least according to Hawking, the robots would threaten to kill, enslave or control all of humanity.

Many Types of Military Robots Emerged

Particularly during the final months of 2015, news reports

described admissions by various governments and corporations on the specific capabilities that scientists were designing for military robots. Among the most unique or notorious of these devices, some in the development stage--while others became far more advanced:

Mine Detection: According to the "Korea Times," South Korean officials were developing specialized robots capable of detecting and removing old explosive mines; this is done in the old Demilitarized Zone between that nation and North Korea.

"Reading Your Mind:" According to the "Defense One" news service, scientists are developing military robots that "can predict your next move." The article was written by Patrick Tucker, the publication's technology editor and author of the book "The Naked Future: What Happens in a World that Anticipates Your Every Move"--an Amazon Best Book of the Month winner in March 2014. Tucker's "Defense One" article said that a 2015 algorithm by two University of Illinois researchers "opens the door to software that can guess where a person is headed--reaching for a gun, steering a car into a armored gate--miliseconds before the act plays out. ... The idea was to help robots help humans, by taking the steering wheel when a driver makes a bad decision, or perhaps activating an exoskeleton when a patient with a weak arm reaches for an object. But the algorithm, broadly speaking, might also help fly a plane or anticipate the next move by a suicide bomber or gunman."

Anti-Killer Robot Movement: According to "Tech Times," opponents of any efforts to develop killer robots and autonomous weapons systems spoke "as a panel" at a press conference held at the United Nations. The global NGO Campaign to Stop Killer Robots contends that governments including the United States are developing the technology much faster than any international effort to legally ban such devices. Yet at least one UN official was quoted as saying that computers can give military and state operations a "split-second advantage"--working much faster than humans. However, as noted by "Tech Times," statistics show that "targeting may not be these potential killer robots' strong points. In a report, nine out of 10 individuals killed by human-controlled drones in Afghanistan during a given five-month period were not the intended targets."

Deadly Varieties Designed

Electricical engineers remained super-busy in early 2016 designing a vast array of robot types for military warfare and clandestine surveillance. Gradually over time, most or all of these new devices will have varying impacts on healthcare worldwide.

Some specific types of these robots were far more advanced than others. Yet various news reports, government press releases and official videos indicated that these were well on the way to full operation. Among those frequently mentioned:

BugBots: As small as natural insects including common houseflies, these machines can enter homes or buildings in large quantities. Just one fly-sized BugBot can generate audio and video recordings of people targeted for surveillance. Most or all of these miniature machines will be able to inject people with deadly poison.

Bird-sized Robots: As small as tiny birds, these machines are designed to perform outdoor surveillance--counting enemy warriors and continually monitoring their locations. Like most advanced robots, these devices continually communicate with each other in battlefield environments--while also sending valuable data to a central command.

Standard Warriors: These machines look like robots, making them easy for adversaries to identify. However, these devices are super-strong and seemingly indestructable, thereby enabling the people who built or operate them to coordinate intense non-stop attacks of targeted communities, human armies or buildings.

Humanoid Warriors: Working alone or in groups, sometimes with human allies, these battling machines look and behave as if real human soldiers--except for one major difference.

Built with super-strength under strict specifications, these devices are seemingly indestructable--destroyed only via nuclear explosions.

Wearable Robots: Human soldiers wear sophisticated robotics parts, which significantly boosts the perceived strength of these people. Humans wearing these machines are sometimes capable of easily running several times faster than an average person, while also possessing vastly superior strength.

Beware of Warlords

While all the various just-mentioned machines are already being tested under simulated battle conditions, officials worry that warlords who manage to steal these machines could use the devices to carry out devilish deeds.

Without question, having and using these super-advanced killing machines might enable people controlling them to eradicate, torture or enslave entire populations.

Under such worst-case scenarios, civilized societies would eventually get obliterated by the same machines that those cultures created to protect themselves.

This generates an inescapable paradox. Although as a whole many types of robots are designed to protect and help society, the same machines ultimately might endanger mankind.

People with average or even typical intelligence could very well become confused or even somewhat "insane" when confronting such inescapable situations. The onslaught of killer robots everywhere seems outside the realm of basic human comprehension, far beyond the abilities of most people to understand or to confront.

Inferior Medical Facility Protection

Worsening all these problems multi-fold, officials including Defense Department administrators seem to have done little or nothing to protect the healthcare system.

Particularly within recent decades, human warriors have

concentrated on targeting and attacking so-called "soft spots," locations that have little or no protection.

Besides crowded trains, jetliners, sports stadiums and theaters, some of the most vulnerable soft spots where lots of people congregate are healthcare facilities like hospitals and medical clinics. Lots of these structures are filled with many people who lack defensive weaponry.

Those infrastructures increases are stuck with the inescapable fact that officials seem to have failed to implement military-style security at those locations.

Attackers could seek to gain an advantage by destroying those facilities, particularly in instances where invaders want to kill as many people as possible.

"Destroying hospitals might be among the best way to kill all of our adversaries," the invaders might tell themselves and their comrades. "Without adequate medical care, most or all of the people that we wound will eventually die."

"Spooky" Outcome Becomes Possible

The race to create deadly robots seems just as dangerous and misguided as the continual efforts to develop advanced medical machines.

Yet here is the "sticking point" that scientists and electrical engineers might be failing to adequately plan for--making "mistakes" when creating the technology.

A proverbial Catch-22 situation results.

You see, from the very start a primary reason for designing, creating and building robots is to eliminate the "mistakes" or "chances for error" that typical humans make.

However, by rushing the design process too fast, people increase the possibility that they will "fail" or make serious "mistakes" in creating the robots.

Once a catastrophe occurs as a direct result of such oversights, it will be too late to "turn back the clock and correct serious problems with programming or design."

Beware of Looming Dangers

The current Rise of Military Robots and the Rise of Medical Robots are the modern equivalent of the 1969 Apollo 11 journey, planned to enable men to walk on the moon for the first time. Back then nearly a half century ago scientists had done their best to minimize or eliminate the possibility of error.

"There will be no second chances for survival on this mission," the general public seemed to be told. "At this point during liftoff from earth, all we can do is know that we have done our very best."

When astronaut Neil Armstrong became the first man to walk on the moon, people celebrated worldwide. But just nine months later in April 1970, the Apollo 13 mission to land more men on the moon experienced a near-fatal catastrophe.

Due to a human-generated design error, an on-board Command Module's oxygen tank exploded two days after liftoff, and while still en route to the moon. Scientists and astronauts at Mission Control on earth worked at a highly creative and furious pace to develop a necessary solution to save the three astronauts on board. Otherwise the trio would have died from an inadequate oxygen supply.

The ability of humans to ingeniously and quickly generate creative solutions to potentially deadly problems sometimes becomes essential.

Tragically, as a result of such human-caused problems, an extreme danger will remain unless humanity generates viable solutions; these situations likely will involve instances where healthcare and military robotics malfunction, on a widespread catastrophic level.

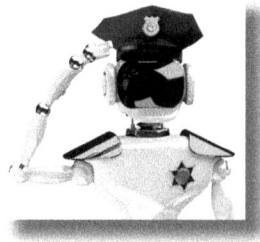

Chapter 35
Welcome to the "Robotics Revolution"

In many ways the current Rise of Robots phenomenon can be compared to the famous Industrial Revolution that drastically changed the world economy nearly 200 years ago.

Between around 1760 to 1840, the advent of machinery for manufacturing drastically changed the typical ways that most people earned their livings.

Before then, practially all merchandise was produced by hand, generally a cumbersome and slow process that bogged down the economy--as most people labored on farms

All that changed thanks to the advent of steam power, water power, and machine tools, plus all-new factory systems that accelerated the production of goods. Largely as a result, many people became motivated to move from farmland to major cities.

Similarly, at least according to some robotics experts, the current rollout of such machines will drastically convert the international economy forever. Once that happens, these experts say, there essentially will be "no turning back, whatsoever."

Use History as a Guide
For thousands of years wise people and those who chronicle societal changes have proclaimed that "history repeats itself." Indeed, every several hundred years for thousands of generations, mankind has devised new methods designed to improve the quality of life.

Right now the latest transition involves automation, primarily involving robots, impacting virtually everything that we "mere humans" do in life.

Virtually everything aspect of the average human life will experience a significant impact, from transportation and communication, to energy, food production, personal security and even ways to wage war--or to help ensure an enduring peace.

By this point, surely you must realize that there is almost no way to avoid such massive change, whether or not we want these transitions to occur. For you and for your family, survival might hinge on the decisions you make now--rather than later.

Instead of fretting over potential job losses caused by such machines, society should "embrace it," according to a CNBC story on the Barclays banking giant's study on the issue--entitled "Future-proofing UK manufacturing."

Propaganda or Truth

At this juncture, even intelligent people could not be blamed if they become confused by such statements--as authorities release diverging opinions of this critical issue. The average person lacks any clue on whether so-called statements by robotics and economics experts are true, or "mere gibberish," concocted to paint an rosy picture.

All along, no matter what "peachy clean" and sparkling stories officials issue regarding the Robotics Revolution, the overall situation had already gotten out of hand regarding the many new technologies.

For instance, with increased intensity heartless and uncaring people began pointing laser beams into the cockpits of commercial airliners. Some aviation experts claimed "it is just a matter of time before a major disaster occurs, as a result of this."

Exacerbating problems even more, people controlling drones reckless flew the aircraft near private aircraft, commercial airliners and even helicopters; these included some instances when crews in those aircraft were battled raging wildfires in remote wildnerness areas.

"People are stupid--at least lots of them are," some observers might proclaim, and rightly so. "Give this type of advanced technology to 100 or 1,000 people, and chances seem high that at least one of them will use the devices to engage in dangerous activity."

Mindless Individuals "Gone Awry"

In much the same way that irresponsible people drink alcohol before driving motor vehicles, many individuals likely will "do the wrong thing" upon getting their hands on new and relatively untested robotics technologies.

The extreme danger here becomes the distinct possibility that even so-called "harmless" robots will become proverbial "ticking time bombs"--at least when owned or handled by people who lack common sense.

The worst of these scenarios very likely could involve almost any sector of the healthcare industry, instances where robots or automated machines interact with patients.

These specific dangers never involve the previously mentioned "hacking issue," but rather people who fail to effectively use the devices--or individuals who refrain from using safety-oriented procedures when managing or manipulating the machines.

An age-old saying based on "Murphy's Law" tells us that "anything that can go wrong, will go wrong." Prime examples involving non-robotic situations included deadly disasters at nuclear power plants. The most famous of these mishaps occurred in 1986 at the Chernobyl Nuclear Power Plant in the Ukraine, and a 2011 tsunami-caused disaster at the Fukushima Daiichi Nuclear Power Plant in Japan.

Assurances of Safety Proved Incorrect

Prior to these nuclear power plant disasters, executives in that industry had essentially given the general public a supposed "100-percent assurance of safety."

These situations emerged as classic examples that "Big Brother" essentially promises everyone that everything will be OK, when in fact the opposite is true.

Well, whether robotics experts and scientists want to hear this or not, any promise that "robots will never get out of hand" should be considered as meaningless.

The many so-called broken promises that people in numerous cultures have been given throughout history are far too numerous to list here in full.

Countless armies have been assured of "certain victories" by their generals and political leaders, before ultimately getting obliterated by their adversaries. Too many people have put their full faith and trust in their so-called leaders.

Increasing the current dangers multi-fold, with steadily increasing frequency in the coming years, people will never know whether the so-called "official messages" that they are receiving on safety are issued by people--or instead by robots.

Envision Worst-Case Scenarios

Mankind's deep fears that robots or Artificial Intelligence might seize control of the world became more apparent than ever in the classic science-fiction narrative, "2001: A Space Odyssey."

First as a short story, "The Sentinel" by Arthur C. Clark, and soon after as a 1968 film directed by Stanley Kubrick, the tale delved into critical issues that still remain highly controversial. Besides Artificial Intelligence and extraterrestrial life, the hot-button themes included human evolution, technology, and existentialism.

Consistently considered by many critics as among the top 10 films of all time, the movie's basic storyline now seems more relevant than ever.

Everything essentially comes down to the burning, non-stop questions that have nagged at the psyches of humans for thousands of years. The pivotal dilemmas involve: who we think we are as humans; where we came from; what role--if any--should technology play in this journey of personal discovery; and what people "should believe in."

Still considered by some people as one of "the greatest films ever made," this classic movie still seems far more relevant now than ever.

In the final scene, without saying so in specific words,

the film delves deep into the critical "essence of how people fit into the universe, the very core of what it means to be a real, live, breathing human being."

In the final scene, after an AI-controlled computer named "Hal" turns off life support in a spacecraft, an astronaut named David Bowman reaches for a black monolith that appears near the foot of his bed. But while trying to grasp the object, Bowman is transformed into a fetus surrounded by a transparent, light-filled orb.

Pivotal Issues Become Evident

Primarily because of the Robot Revolution, with steadily increasing intensity people today are being confronted by the same issues that Bowman encountered.

Besides reflecting on their own religions and the so-called "meaning of life," more than ever before today's humans must question the usefulness and need for technology.

Perhaps most distressing, whether or not we want to admit this, average people are needing to reflect on the previously mentioned issues involving Artificial Intelligence.

"All these details keep swarming into our brains, even those of us with average IQs," I tell people who ask me about these pivotal details. "Every person must confront these issues head-on, rather than just those of us who fashion ourselves as intellectuals."

Yes, we have reached a pivotal juncture in human history, at a precise point where robotics and AI will lead to the much-feared destruction of humanity--or toward the betterment of mankind as a whole.

Entering an Actual "Brave New World"

These many disturbing factors point to the irreversable and undenial fact that society is litterally entering a "Brave New World," reminiscient of the classic 1931 novel by that name written by Aldous Huxley.

Eerly predicting today's many technologies, Huxley's eternal classic delved into such contentious issues as sleep learning, psychological manipulation, and reproductive technology. Often ranked among the best English language novels of the 20th Century, the book delves into many of the same issues emerging due to the Robot Revolution.

"This might sound eerily spooky or strange, but human beings often have an uncanny ability to envision the destructive challenges resulting from technology," I sometimes say. "As for robots, we just need to look into our hearts to see the disturbing truth. And, when we do that, our hearts and souls might become understandably terrified."

Indeed, this is no laughing matter. Essentially, due to the increasingly rapid Rise of the Robots, all of humanity is essentially becoming the proverbial "guinea pig for scientists, literally a laboratory test mouse."

Jarring our emotional senses and our God-given psyches even more, at this pivotal juncture in human history there is no way for us to undo the advancements in robotics. Both sad and tragic, our current situation is enough to leave humanity breathless, somewhat incapable of putting our sense of loss into discernable words.

Allow Eternal Wisdom to Endure

Many of history's wisest people have consistently taught society that the greatest enduring pathway to a peaceful eternity is love.

From Gautama Buddah to Jesus Christ and several others, this essential message has been enduring and powerful enough to pass down through the ages.

Now, more than ever before the need for love and for empathy toward all humanity is more essential than ever, particularly as robots spread worldwide.

Everything comes down to the pivotal fact that we as human beings deserve to maintain and thrive without unnatural machines, just as Mother Nature has intended.

To deny this essential factor would be to turn our backs on who we are, both individually and collectively.

Indeed, what we have on our own without the nuts, bolts, wires, metals and plastics of machines is the essence of life. Our minds, souls and motivations hail as precious, irreplaceable and worthy of saving forevermore.

Never Acquiesce to Robotics

Cognizant of the burning need to save humanity from itself, we should never acquiesce to the Rise of the Robots.

To enable and allow machines to seize control of every aspect of society, to give in to their instructions and to surrender our creativity to them is an ultimate sin.

Yes, a sin is anything or any behavior that rips away at the very fabric of what it means to be a human being. What we're talking about here is the Golden Rule often mentioned by spiritual leaders, "Do unto others, as you would have them do unto you."

Yet conversely what is "right and correct" to do in different situations is a matter of argument. Some scientists might argue that the loving and caring thing to do would be to create robots that "help us" and "replace us"--while others might argue otherwise.

Such spiritual and philosophical contrasts bring to mind another age-old saying that suddenly become more essential than ever--"Beware of a wolf in sheep's clothing," because otherwise you might get murdered, captured, tortured, brainwashed, enslaved, and eaten.

Beware of Scientists With So-Called "Good Intentions"

Wary of others who have betryed them in the past, or still fully cognizant of lessons taught by their parents long ago, lots of people today sometimes proclaim that "the road to hell is sometimes paved with good intentions."

The internationally acclaimed physicist Albert Einstein, whose discoveries led to the creation of the nuclear bomb, once said: "I know not with what weapons World War III will be fought, but World War IV will be fought with sticks and stones."

Such disturbing and insightful observations help underscore the inescapable fact that mankind keeps heading down a precarious road, particularly if we continue allowing robotics advancements to surge forward without regulations or sensible oversight.

Nonetheless, a disturbing factor enters deep into the heart of this issue, the supposed need or desire by some societies to "be the first at significant robotics advancements"--rather than risk destruction from those who would do so first.

"The principle of self defense, even involving weapons and bloodshed, has never been condemned--even by Ghandi," said the Rev. Dr. Martin Luther King Jr., the famed U.S. civil rights activist, famed for his pacifist approach to making positive change.

Show Courage: Display Your Emotions

"If we were to lose the ability to be emotional, if we were to lose the ability to be angry, to be outraged, we would be robots. And I refuse that," said Suzanna Arundhati Roy, an Indian author and winner of the 1997 Man Booker Prize for Fiction.

Latching on to this essential issue, streams of other notable internationally famous celebrities have also unabashedly voiced their many criticisms about robotics. Individually and collectively, they describe the Robot Revolution as a push-pull or ying-yang situation, where virtually no one seems to emerge as a "true" winner.

"We humans have a love-hate relationship with our technology," said Daniel H. Wilson, a "New York Times" best-selling author and robotics engineer. "We love each new advance, and we hate how fast our world is changing ... The robots really embody that love-hate relationship we have with technology."

Ripping a huge and potentially destructive swath deep into the essence of this issue, some people also openly talk about what they perceive as the beautiful, glorious and stupendous process of building robots that are creative.

Reggie Watts, an American actor, singer and musician, has been quoted as saying that "as a child I was very into gadgets and machines and robots. The idea of experimenting with machines to create art was always something I tinkered with."

The Differences Between "Right and Wrong"

Compounding these challenges multi-fold, the Robot Revolution involves far more than merely programming certain moral and value systems into the machines--an issue briefly mentioned earlier.

Besides merely coding or ordering the machines on "how to behave or what to do," society as a whole needs to grasp the difficult-to-differentiate fact that all humans have different perspectives on what is "right or wrong."

Millions or even billions of people might think that it's perfectly OK to build and distribute highly creative robots--while just as many others could very well argue otherwise. All along, society increasingly finds itself needing to confront these issues head-on, full-force due to the Information Age made possible by the Internet.

Almost everyone worldwide has the instant ability to learn about many new technologies as soon as those advancements emerge. This proverbial puzzle continually becomes more complex, as new devices stream into the consumer marketplace; all this happens seemingly much faster than an average person would have time to mentally absorb and fully assimilate such changes.

"This is a far contrast from several thousand years ago, when all average people needed to know was how to get food and shelter--the mere basics," I sometimes tell my colleagues. "By sharp contrast, in today's world, no single person could ever possibly know or mentally grasp all the many changes that have occurred--or will occur soon."

Locked in a Non-Stop Ferris Wheel

Due to these countless technological advancements, virtually every man, woman and child in today's industrialized nations is essentially "locked in a non-stop Ferris wheel." Collectively and individually, we continually go up and down on a proverbial sphere--the device that carries us always changing due continuous technological advancements.

At least in a hypothetical sense, none of us can hop off of this maze, since the Internet--and increasingly robotics as well--are controlling every aspect of our lives.

Oh, sure, as individuals, families and entire cultures, we can choose to ignore or avoid robotics and the Web. But such endeavors would fail to take away the fact that these infrastructures ultimately control every basic life necessity, from food to energy.

"I envision a time when we will be to robots what dogs are to humans, and I'm rooting for the machines," said Claude Elwood Shannon, an American electronic engineer, hailed as the "Father of Information Theory;" he died in Massachusetts in 2001 at age 84.

Shannon's disturbing forecasts strike many people as ominious, particulalry as robots steadily edge into almost every aspect of our daily lives.

Everything Changes in the Blink of an Eye

Whether we want to admit this or not, the many changes made possible by robotics are seemingly occurring "within the blink of an eye."

All the world's greatest minds and even super-computers likely have varying and sharply diverging opinions on how we should react.

"If you look at the field of robotics today, you can say robots have been in the deepest oceans, they've been to Mars, you know?" said Cynthia Lynn Breazeal, an associate professor of Media Arts and Sciences at the Massachusetts Institute of Technology. "They've been all these places, but they're just now starting to come into your living room. Your living room is the final frontier of robots."

Such comments bring to mind yet another great American novel, the eternal 1949 classic "Nineteen Eighty Four"--sometimes published as "1984" and written by widely acclaimed writer George Orwell. The plot features a superstate called "Airstrip One," in a state of perpetual war.

Like many people interacting with robots today, the characters in "1984" need to deal with what seems to them as an invented language. Even more disturbingly, that fictional society mirrors what many citizens must endure today, continual government monitoring of all communications.

Government Intrusion Worsens

Eerily like the plots of "1984," "Brave New World," and "2001: A Space Odyssey," government intrusion into the personal lives of everyday citizens is likely to worsen due to the Robot Revolution.

Besides continually monitoring your healthcare and personal behavior, advanced robots likely will track the movements of every person within industrialized countries.

Adding a disturbing level of horror to this mix, scientists might very well have the aforementioned capability of either "reading your thoughts" or sending information into your mind. All this would be done by surgically implanted microchips.

Legendary American political activist and anarchist Abbie Hoffman eerily commented on the issue, long before most people even realized the Rise of the Robots would happen.

"Become an internationalist and learn to respect all life. Make war on machines--in particular the sterile machines of corporate death and the robots that guard them," said Hoffman, who committed suicide in 1989 at age 52.

Some People Take an Opposite Approach

In keeping with basic human nature, other intellectuals in

recent decades have sharply disagreed with or avoided any efforts to launch anti-robot protests.

Among those championing and pushing hard for what they describe as reasonable advancements in robotics is Kenneth Y. Goldberg, an American researcher in that industry who also works as a writer, inventor and artist.

Credited for his 1994 creation of the first robot with a Web interface, alone or with his students Goldberg has authored at least 170 peer-review technical papers on algorithms for social information filtering, automation and robotics.

Also a leading researcher in "cloud robotics" and the aforementioned telerobotics, he has been quoted as saying that "our robots are signing up for online learning. After decades of attempts to program robots to perform complex tasks like flying helicopters and surgical surturing, the new approach is based on observing and recording the motions of human experts as they perform these feats."

Scientific visionaries and robotics industry entrepreneurs are likely to embrace such efforts on a broad scale. This ideology would conflict with people who finally will protest once they discover what some will claim as "the heart literally being ripped out of the very essence of humanity--all because of mere machines."

Established Philosophies Obliterated

Eventually reaching a proverbial "maddening level," the building of a firmly established international robotics infrastructure would wreak havoc on many of mankind's basic philosophies, some established several hundred years before Christ.

The famous Greek philosopher Socrates, his widely acclaimed pupil Plato and Aristotle collectively and individually created a philosophy grounded by mathematics and science. Eventually becoming Aristotle's teacher, Plato has often been acclaimed as a founder of Western religion and spirituality.

"A good decision is based on knowledge and not on

numbers," said Plato, his philosophy here in direct conflict with what now has become the robotics industry--a field in which basic and essential algorithms depend on digital-based numbers.

Just as haunting was Plato's observation that "one of the penalties for refusing to participate in politics is that you end up being governed by your inferiors."

The irony here emerges from the inescapable fact that many of today's brightest minds fear that robots could eventually seize the decision-making process--a creepy observation made possible by the fact that politicians have failed to regulate robotics.

Anticipate Government Failures

Some historians argue that every government and political ideology since the earliest recorded civilizations has had serious flaws, failures and corruption.

Many dynasties or empires have disappeared during the past 3,000 years, often because their adversaries developed better technologies and weaponry.

The current dangers here are potentially more catastrophic than those of the past, amid a whirlwind of deadly and seemingly unstoppable tragedies.

Besides floods and droughts that caused food shortages in many underdeveloped countries, domestic and international terrorism surged into the late 2010s.

This likely movitated the world's handful of remaining superpowers to drastically accelerate the development of advanced robotic weaponry and defense systems.

All this occurred in a "perfect storm," amid riots or heated disputes involving conflicting idiologies involving race, political philosophies and income inequality.

Dangers of Worldwide Conflict Increased

The international culture loaded with these many differences reached a proverbial "boiling point," by the beginning of 2016.

As robotics research and developments intensified at an unprescedented pace, tensions increased among the three superpowers--the United States, Russia and China.

Any sense of logic or efforts to push for peace seemed as if swept by the wayside, while these adversaries seemed to position themselves for potential full-scale war.

Needless to say, the need and demand for protective robots intensified, particularly within the U.S.A. as a response to various shooting attacks on innocent people. By the end of 2015, robots were mentioned in news reports on almost a weekly basis, the devices used to locate or to eliminate potential explosives left by assailants.

Meanwhile, the growing number of wounded from such attacks seemed to sharply increase the demand or need for super-sophisticated medical robots.

Robots to the Rescue?

The mere mention of robots seemed to impress some people as sensible and even logical, eliminating the need for police and soldiers to unnecessarily risk their lives.

Meantime, the international and domestic infrastructure became endangered, as if a pent-up kettle ready to blow into a cataclysm of seemingly indescribable proportions.

These various factors, in turn, generated two opposing or conflicting views regarding robots, inescapable details that officials needed to consider:

Helpful: Under this ideology, high-functioning robots are needed fast to essentially "save mankind from itself, thereby rescuing everyone in the process."

Hurtful: From this perspective, robots can and will do far more harm than good, endangering humanity--while also robbing people everywhere of their liberties.

Expect Drastic Changes Worldwide

Whether positive or negative, officials within the scientific and military communities seemed to agree that "life for all mankind was about to change forever."

An "inconvenient truth" emerged, namely the inescapable fact that robots were to play a significant role.

From at least one disturbing perspective, the citizens of the world were about to attend a theoretical "shotgun wedding."

Under this scenario the groom would be robotics, machines and any advanced technology; the bride is the delicate and vulnerable condition of humanity, left with no option other than to put all of its full faith, hope and trust in its intended new spouse.

Yet sadly, even before these hypothetical nuptials commenced, deep down in their hearts people seemed to know that this would emerge as a dysfunctional marriage.

Robotics and Humanity:
The "Ultimate Dysfunctional" Couple

In my view, following many years of study and in-depth research into these critical issues, the full blending and coupling of robotics and humanity form the "ultimate dysfunctional couple." Quite disturbingly, people and AI-enhanced machines are becoming co-dependent on one another.

This blending of nature with the "unreal" is essentially creating a bond that--when together--creates an inescapable and destructive paradox.

To put this situation into perspective, think of any dysfunctional and co-dependant real-life husband and wife that you have undoubtedly met.

The intermixing of humans with advanced robots forms the kind of couple that "cannot live with each other, and they cannot live without each other either."

Herein rests what Shakespeare, the greatest English-language writer in world history, would call "The Rub." Indeed, humanity has reached a pivotal sticking point, an urgent historical juncture that likely will determine the mankind's fate.

The Ultimate Question: "To Be, or Not to Be?"

Shakespeare's world-famous sililoquy by Hamlet, the famous "to be, or not to be" line comes to mind when considering mankind's dilemma involving robotics.

Under one way of thinking, to be without robots is to embrace nature as the Creator intended; conversely, being with the machines is devilish, unnatural and destructive.

Another philosophy appreciates and adores everything that involves robots, while the thought of being without them seems unnatural and catastrophic. This asserts that mankind cannot be trusted to live and thrive on its own.

Such disputes fail to remove the fact that the eternally iconic Shakespearan speech delves into the very essence of human nature. Particularly when factoring robotics into the mix, the many lines and phrases from this speech take on a freaky nature.

Terms ranging from "what dreams may come" to the "dread of something after death" seem to take on whole new meanings--either treacherous or angelic.

Are Illuminati Fears Merely Absurd?

Many people fearing mankind's potential dependence on robots fear that such technologal advancements are part of a devilish scheme to create a New World Order.

While some observers label such fears as "mere nonsense," others insist that the world's richest people are secretly working to create a single international government.

To help carry out this scheme, the world's richest people called the "illuminati" would use robots to control the behaviors, movements and freedoms of everyone.

Perceptions regarding such supposed international conspiracies are sometimes viewed as over-the-top fears voiced by "political whackos." Critics label people who worry about the New World Order as paranoid schizophrenics.

However, such observations have failed to dissuade the "believers," some who produced compelling online videos that protrayed President Barack Obama as a champion of efforts to create a socialist-dominated New World Order.

The Disappearance of National Borders

Such a "one-world, and one-nation" philosophy envisions a world without borders, a universal society in which people come and go as they please without any bounderies between--what until now--society has viewed as independent countries.

As a key example of this, critics cite the fact that Obama refrained from aggressively attacking radical Islamic terrorists, particularly during 2015. Throughout Europe at the time many socialist-leaning, liberal national leaders also embraced a "no-borders" ideology.

These whacky and illogical political philosophies came into question when millions of immigrants streamed from war-torn Syria into Europe.

Then, in the wake of a horrific attack on November 13, 2015, radical Islamic terrorists in Paris slaughtered more than 129 people. In the immediate aftermath, police discovered evidence that some of the attackers were Islamists who had migrated from Syria into Greece.

The perceived need for high-functioning robots suddenly intensified as a result. Such machines were used to protect police officers investigating the crime scenes, and also when authorities attacked a suspected stronghold or hideout used by the terrorists.

Were Fears Unfounded or Legitimate?

Was it true that Obama and his socialist allies worldwide secretly encouaged or "looked the other way"--all in hopes that the terrorism and massive human migration would lead to a New World Order? Also, and just as disturbingly, could this have been part of a long-term strategy to make people feel more reliant and dependent on robots?

If true, such a warped and devilish political ideology would mirror the creepy transformation of China. That nation gradually transformed its government away from the ideology of Mao Zedong, Chairman of the Communist Party of China from its 1949 inception until his 1976 death.

Essentially, today's China equals a creepy mix of communism and capitalism, where an elite handful of rulers are extremely rich--while controlling and limiting the speech, freedoms and activities of its impoverished general citizenry.

In a sense, this system mirrors an ideology that critics claim is embraced by Obama, his socialist allies and their cohorts pushing for a New World Order.

Even if such fears are unfounded, ludicrous or over-the-top, at least one critical factor has become undeniable.

Yes, robots and the continual creation and development of such machines shall continue from this point forward, at least until becoming incapable of doing that.

So, the fate of humanity likely will rest in decisions made by people building the devices, and--most disturbingly--perhaps even eventually by the machines.

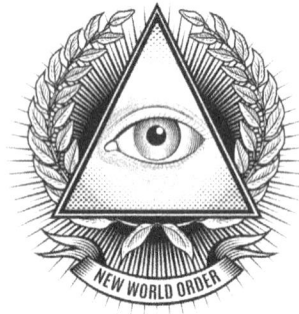

Chapter 36
Stop the Lunacy! Ban RoboDocs Now

Perhaps the biggest shock to the human psyche comes the revelation that fully autonomous RoboDocs could become prevalent in healthcare within 20 to 30 years.

The very notion of such machines should be enough to strike fear and trepidation into the hearts and minds of any person who learns about such efforts.

This becomes particularly disturbing, when considering the fact that anti-killer robot protests have emerged worldwide in recent years; amazingly, this has happened without an anti-RoboDoc demonstrations being reported anywhere in the world.

Such a disturbing oversight likely has happened due to the basic fact that--at least until the point of this book's publication, most people had remained oblivious to this urgent issue.

"What we fail to know can sometimes kill us," I sometimes say. "Having advanced robotic doctors developed without your knowledge, is almost like having a cancer grow throughout your body for many years--without you ever knowing."

Unless programmed, built and used in a reasonable manner, RoboDocs could emerge just as deadly and destructive to humans as military robots. Both types of machines could individually and collectively lead to tens of millions of deaths.

Delving into Dangerous Theory

At present, electrical engineers might insist that the general public would have absolutely nothing to fear from any type of medical robot--particularly RoboDocs.

Such declarations might seem well-intentioned when viewed "at face value."

Even so, a sad, horrible and inescapable revelation emerges from the fact that destructive robotic doctors easily might have any or all of the many flaws already described.

Besides the aforementioned security oversights such as hackers, inept politicians without any medical knowledge are likely to dictate how RoboDocs are programmed.

Worsening matters multi-fold becomes the previously mentioned fact that mainstream medicine might control this process, thereby requiring that high-level medical robots be programmed to prescribe dangerous BigPharma drugs in all instances.

"The world's industrialized nations are essentially playing Russian Roulette with each of our lives, particularly if they allow such technologies to move foward without strict regulation," any reasonable person could say. "Worst of all, once this infrastructure is set into place, there literally could be no turning back--whatsoever."

Legitimate Reasons for Fear

As distrubing as this seems, the general public has a right to become concerned and even fearful. Also, remember the aforementioned fact that authorities have an extreme motivation--namely tremdous profits.

This means that you, your family and everyone you know will get targeted in the crosshairs of this giant transformation. To say that there is an "organized conspiracy" to overthrow and control the entire healthcare industry would be an exaggeration.

However, officials cannot erase the fact that this "race to be the best, cutting-edge medical services" is well underway. Unless something is done to stop this nonsense, consumers could suddenly become endangered due to the "disappearance of human doctors."

When and if that happens, humanity likekly will have lost any hope for its survival, at least any form of human being that we have known until now.

Yes, we as people have a right and duty to voice our grave concerns. To do otherwise--to allow robots and AI to permeate the entire healthcare industry--would rob humanity of "the very essence of what it means to be a human being."

Listen to Your Heart and Soul

Put all these diverging factors into clear perspective by sitting alone in a quiet place. Close your eyes and breathe deeply for several minutes.

Throughout this process, strive to clear your mind of distracting thoughts about your family. Avoid thinking about your personal finances, daily obligations, sensitive matters and any other issue that invariably clutters your thoughts.

Ideally when doing this, you also might play a soothing recording, such as the gentle sound of waves continually cascading on a beach or the noise of barely discernable crickets.

Even better, engage in this meditative process outdoors in the middle of the night, far away from the noise, lights and craziness of city life.

Perhaps over multiple sessions of repeating this process, with persistance and careful planning over time, you eventually will put your mind into a clear place. When that happens, begin contemplating a world filled with RoboDocs and mechanical nurses.

You very likely will discover an important message delivered straight to your mind by your heart and soul; each of us instinctively knows the "truth" about humanity, Mother Nature and the eternal need for people to benefit from nature whenever possible.

Humans are Important

Yes, your heart and soul can tell you clearly and forcefully what the mind often refuses to convey. Everything comes down to the inescapable fact that humans have been given a unique place within the universe by our Creator.

Whatever your religion or spiritual belief might be, the heart will tell you that each of us has been given a special gift in this regard.

Our ability to create, to love, to cry, to think, and to undergo failures, successes and disappointments helps make us who we are today.

This life that we have is a gift for all the ages, a blessed miracle that we need to nurture and to protect--both now and for all subsequent generations.

Those of us who choose to be agnostics or athiests can and should realize that we all posess an innate ability to love--and that means doing our best to separate or divorce humanity from invasive, distructive robotic inventions.

Expect an Onslaught of Propaganda

Common sense tells us that many books, magazines, TV shows and movies will be produced on this essential topic-- particularly during the next few decades.

Fully cognizant of this likely scenario well beforehand, you can now begin to prepare yourself mentally for this confusing propaganda.

Powerful business interests that control and have a financial interest in robots in all likelihood will strive to push a maze of misinformation into the brains of the public.

"Robots are the new miracle of today," we will be told. "Healthcare machines are among the best! Yes, isn't this amazing! As people, we no longer have to make critical choices regarding our own health. These phenomenal machines do all that for us!"

While such information might seem like "pure nonsense," at least based on current media accounts, this horrific type of informational deception could soon become a "reality."

Stay Strong and Remain Motivated

In whatever way that these many technological advances progress, you need to remain physically and mentally strong-- while encouraging your family to do the same.

With equal importance, amid every step of this disturbing transition, you and everyone that you know should remain motivated to keep humanity viable and essential.

For instances involving the healthcare industry, each of us needs to take the following peaceful and decisive actions:

Avoidance: Refuse to use the services of any hospital or medical clinic that uses RoboDocs, particularly facilities that ban or refuse to employ human physicians.

Strength: Remain mindful that an age-old saying remains true, "there is strength in numbers." Use this strategy to join with other people in collectively opposing the full saturation of medical robots into the entire mainstream healthcare industry.

Corruption: Always remain aware that politicians, BigPharma and federal bureaucracies dealing with health care are generally corrupt and self-serving. Thus, there is little that can be done to prevent them from encouraging and clearing the way for the massive rollout of medical robots--all in an effort to save money.

Go Natural: While avoiding robotic healthcare and human physicians allied to this transition, in whatever way reasonably possible, you should seek the services of Homeopaths, Naturopaths and other human healthcare professionals highly trained in natural remedies.

Natural Medicines: Require that medical robots factor in essential and sensible natural medicines into their treatment protocols. Robots and AI machines should always use natural substances as a preferred method over unnatural, dangerous, expensive and addictive drugs produced by BigPhrama.

Self-Help: Take a pro-active approach to your own health, and encourage your relatives or loved ones to do the same. This means using common sense as a motivation to exercise in moderation, while eating and resting in as healthy a way as possible.

End Obamacare: Legally obliterate the tragic and destructive Obamacare regulations, particularly the bureaucratic sector in which people without any medical training make critical decisions regarding the healthcare industry. This would be possible only through "the power of the ballot box."

"Tax Them" Heavily: Even those of us who are fiscally and politically conservative should consider the enactment of a heavy, huge tax on the medical robotic industry--particularly any firm that produces RoboDocs. These revenues should be sent directly to every U.S. citizen, as compensation for the "emotional pain" and mental suffering that each of us would have to endure under such a healthcare infrastructure.

Food Industry Regulation: One of the most essential health-related issues involes the production and distrubiton of crops and animals used for food. With steadily increasing intensity in recent years, major corporations have won governmental approval to use automated or robotic systems to produce or genetically modify our food. Particularly as robots become an increasingly essential part of that process, consumers should push for regulations to: ban genetically modified food (GMOs); require that the packaging of GMO foods be clearly labeled as having that attribute; require labeling that specifies where and how each food product is produced; and criminalize the use of machines to prepare and serve restaurant meals-- specifically instances that would remove people from the process.

Medical Schools: Enact a nationwide federal law that: bans the use of tele-instructors in medical schools; requires that human professors and doctors teach students; requires that these institutions offer courses that stress the essential need to make human doctors a required part of all healthcare institutions.

Robot Clubs and Classes: Require that all robot clubs and classes at high schools and colleges have at least some essential instruction on "the vital need to keep humans in the process"--particularly endeavors involving health care.

Hacking Concerns: When regulating medical robots and machines used for other industries, require that the manufacturers have installed or implement effective anti-hacking attributes; these anti-hack coding procedures or digital platforms would serve as a vital safety feature in protecting patients from those with harmful intentions.

Minimize Dependence: Authorities must prevent or criminalize the implentation of any healthcare system that would make patients fully dependent on machines. This means keeping human beings specializing in medicine as an essential part of the healthcare process; as a result, patients would "still have a chance if all robots break, or the manufacturers of those machines go bankrupt."

Disturbing Summary

Ultimately, all of society needs to take a far greater "common-sense approach" to the implementation of medical robots.

For the sake of ourselves, our children and grandchildren, at this relatively early stage in this change we must take positive and decisive action.

Otherwise, the many sensible and helpful characteristics of the entire healthcare industry will soon become "a thing of the past."

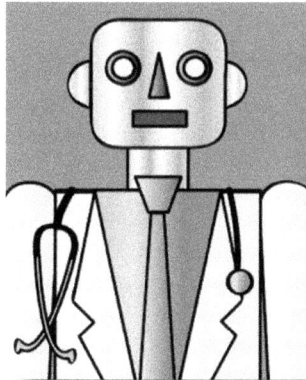

My Clinic's Vastly Superior Survival Rate

The five-year survival rate of advanced Stage IV cancer patients treated at my clinic is nearly 33 times better than the national average.

On a nationwide basis only a dismal 2.1 percent of all such patients survive after being treated by mainstream oncologists who deliver high-dose standard chemo.

By comparison, results at my Century Wellness clinic reflect a 5-year survival rate of more than 71 percent among such patients that I had treated at the time of this book's publication.

To put this into clear perspective, think of the situation this way: only two out of 100 advanced-stage cancer patients survive when treated by conventional cancer doctors. In sharp contrast, at least 71 out of every 100 similar people survive when I treat them. There are several reasons:

Unique tests: My clinic offers chemosensitivity tests that determine which types of chemo will most effectively treat a specific individual, while also identifying which drugs, hormones and natural supplements work best for the patient.

Effective process: Before treatment begins, I meet with each patient to develop an effective treatment process based largely on results of the chemosensitivity tests.

Natural treatments: My clinic uses effective and safe natural treatments that not only refrain from damaging the body, while killing cancer and fortifying their natural immunity. These are unlike dangerous drugs used by mainstream oncologists who often administer harmful synthetic substances that destroy the patient's health and may lead to death.

Cancer obliterated: In most cases my unique treatments generate a 90-plus-percent kill rate of the cancers within such patients. This often enables the patients' immune systems to assume and to successfully carry out the job of completing our fight against the disease, leading to remission. The natural ability of my patients to kill off all remaining cancer increases significantly when I administer superior, effective immune-boosting natural substances.

The 71-percent cancer survival rate generated by Century Wellness Clinic reflects patients who will remain alive five years after treatment. Some survivors at that point may have at least some cancer; among many of these individuals the disease is considered "manageable." Most doctors generally refer to such patients as "cured," particularly individuals who remain in remission after five years.

Consider Me Unique

My treatments sharply boost the possibility of a cure, thanks to the fact that the chemosensitivity tests specify which drugs would work best, and which would be ineffective for each specific patient.

As noted in my newsletters for patients, thanks to the chemosensitivity tests made possible by genomics research, "no other oncologist in the United States can offer this kind of information to his or her patients. What conventional oncologists offer only is what has been the best results of the latest clinical study."

Those reports, which have nothing to do with chemosensitivity tests fail to generate 85-percent accuracy. In fact, many studies embraced by mainstream oncologists are only 30 percent to 50 percent successful.

Results show that conventional chemotherapy treatments administered by mainstream oncologists would never help one half to two thirds of Stage IV cancer patients.

Sadly, these patients are merely being poisoned when given chemotherapy, which does nothing to eliminate cancer-- while intensifying their suffering.

Consider Me A Maverick Doctor

Before initially visiting my clinic, many patients soon realize that I'm one of just a handful of working "integrative medical oncologists" worldwide.

This means that I'm fully licensed to practice medicine as a mainstream medical oncologist, while simultaneously working as a board-certified Homeopathic physician using natural treatments.

• "I essentially use what some people call 'the best of both medical worlds,'" I sometimes tell patients. "If I'm giving you the wrong drug, I'm killing you. But that's what traditional oncologists are doing every day."

My unique Century Wellness Clinic, located in Reno, Nevada, in the western United States, fights cancer with harmless and effective natural substances. We do this without the excessive use of the poisonous, dangerous and expensive drugs such as high-dose chemo administered by mainstream oncologists.

Instead, depending on each patient's specific needs and results of the person's chemosensitivity tests, I develop individualized treatment regimens. These often include extremely limited regimens of low-dose chemo along with various natural remedies.

Sadly, mainstream oncologists are forced by the standard medical industry's required protocol to administer deadly regimens of high-dose chemo to all advanced Stage IV cancer patients--with no exceptions.

From the view of many mainstream doctors, I'm threatening to "overturn the proverbial apple cart."

Under such a scenario, would the resulting "public outcry" generate an ideal situation where frustrated patients worldwide and vote-hungry politicians insist that every mainstream oncologist order chemosensitivity tests for all cancer patients?

Patients Yearn for Effective Natural Remedies

Every week streams of patients from around the world travel to Century Wellness Clinic for treatment of cancer or other ailments.

Every week out-of-state license plates are seen in my clinic's parking lot, after patients drive from as far away as Maine, Florida, Alaska, Canada and Mexico.

This influx of visitors provides a consistent and significant boost to the Reno-area economy, generating thousands of hotel room occupancy, with average patient stays at three to four weeks.

A noticeable portion of these patients from every continent except Antarctica. courageously visit my clinic, after being told by mainstream oncologists elsewhere tell to get their affairs in order.

"Never take the word of any doctor who would tell you something like that," I say to patients. "Every patient needs to remain hopeful for as long as possible."

Genetics Research Makes this Possible

Much of Century Wellness Clinic's success in effectively treating cancer patients has been made possible by genomics research, along with my previously mentioned natural remedies.

These technological advances stem from studies inspired by the Human Genome Project, when scientists mapped out the entire human genome from 1990 to 2003.

Findings made possible by genomic research since then have enabled scientists to develop the amazing chemosensitivity tests. I consider this as an essential, vital and necessary tool for cancer doctors when developing effective individual treatment regimens. Yet keep in mind that as previously mentioned, mainstream oncologists insist on ignoring these techniques.

So, as you might imagine, I've been called a "maverick doctor," largely due to my unwillingness to follow the proverbial dictates of allopathic physicians.

You see, I refrain from "following the proverbial pack" of mainstream doctors. Instead, I choose to essentially stand in my own field while proudly enabling my patients to benefit from effective new genomic technologies that other doctors ignore.

Patients Benefit From Choices

My Stage IV cancer patients at Century Wellness Clinic are given a choice regarding their own treatment regimens.

This serves as a sharp contrast from the process offered by mainstream oncologists; those physicians refuse to enable patients to make such decisions.

At my clinic, patients who wish to go conventional at least know about the best drugs for them. At that point, they then have the right answer. We also offer low-dose (10%-15%) insulin-potentiated chemotherapy over a three-week period.

We also send all patients home with the appropriate supplements deemed highly effective for their individual cancers, renewing these products on an as-needed monthly basis.

Chemosensitivity Testing Works Wonders

Every year, tens of thousands or perhaps millions of cancer patients in the United States fail to receive genomics-generated cancer chemosensitivity tests that could save their lives.

In countless instances such procedures could prevent certain patients from receiving poisonous chemo that never would help them. When that happens high-dose chemo ravages their bodies. This invariably leads to extremely painful, horrendous and lingering death. Their bodies literally waste away.

"On a widespread social scale, this is a tragedy seemingly beyond belief," I tell patients who inquire about the issue. "The sad fact is that most mainstream oncologists either refuse to or fail to inform their patients that chemosensitivity tests exist."

From the standpoint of the vast majority of allopathic cancer doctors, everything essentially comes down to "guesswork" because of the dismal fact that they refrain from seeking such procedures.

Compounding the problem, as mentioned earlier, medical industry standards require mainstream oncologists to follow "protocol." These puzzling rules mandate that all patients with certain types of advanced-stage cancers always be given specific full-dose types of chemo drugs at a pre-designated, high-level; these are administered on pre-set schedules.

Disturbing Results Emerged

By my estimates, in the United States every day nationwide more than 1,300 cancer patients needlessly die such deaths--the equivalent of several jumbo jets crashing into the ocean.

The amount of human suffering is immeasurable on a grand scale.

Yet why do mainstream doctors refuse to recommend such tests? Does mainstream medicine's close ties with Big Pharma--the giant multi-billion-dollar pharmaceutical industry--have anything to do with such the disturbing behavior of these physicians on a grand scale?

While no one can accurately give an irrefutable answer to these critical questions, at least something is clear--patients need to be proactive.

Demand Such Tests

Any person suffering from cancer, particularly advanced Stage IV levels of the disease, should demand the option of taking such tests before any chemo begins. Here are the steps such patients should take:

Access: Before treatment begins, tell the doctor that you want a "cancer chemosensitivity test."

Options: Inquire about what options are available from the doctor for receiving such tests.

History: Ask if the doctor has ever given patients access to such procedures.

Red Flags: Be on the lookout for a "red-flag warning" that if the physician refuses to offer these tests.

Avoid Conventional Oncologists

When I tell my clinic's cancer patients about this, they

immediately start avoiding mainstream oncologists--often telling many people that they know to do the same.

I have been issuing such warnings for many years.

In fact, as I noted in my clinic's October 2010 newsletter, "gene testing has the answers" for cancer patients seeking to benefit from cutting-edge technology.

From my view now in my fifth decade of practicing cancer medicine, the development of such tests emerged as "the biggest C-change in all my years of practice with more than 200,000 patient visits."

Patients Appreciate Access

At Century Wellness Clinic, the advent of cancer chemosensitivity testing has made a major difference in the lives of our patients' success levels and improved overall survival rates. These statistics became evident in our present, ongoing 6-year, 1,000-patient study.

Drawing whole blood at my clinic, cancer chemosensitivity tests are relatively simple, easy and productive procedures. Upon their initial visits to Century Wellness, some people with cancer are what homeopaths call "virginal treatment patients."

The designation signifies that those individuals have not yet been treated for their cancers, and therefore have never been subjected to potentially dangerous or deadly treatments such as multiple drugs, radiation, or even major surgery.

For the most part upon their initial visits to Century Wellness, these patients know that their disease is advancing, and their prognosis is guarded. They know their time factors are limited and they want real answers, along with effective non-toxic treatment.

Avoid the Guessing Game

Most of them highly educated and extremely inquisitive, these patients want to avoid getting ensnared in the type of "guessing game" used by mainstream oncologists.

With equal importance, as I clearly stated in my 2010 newsletter, these patients "don't want an oncologist that picks out drugs and throws them against a wall to see if any stick in terms of their own cancer response rates."

A highly trained and experienced member of my professional staff begins the chemosensitivity testing process by taking a patient's whole blood--a very simple and easy procedure. The blood is then handled very carefully, while undergoing stringent packaging and shipping requirements; samples remain good for 96 hours prior the time when the Greek laboratory analyzes the sample.

My personnel always draw the blood on the first part of the week, ensuring that the sample gets to its destination in a safe, preserved and fresh manner.

Upon arrival at the testing laboratory, scientists and lab technicians subject the blood to high-tech tests. At last count, my clinic estimated that at least three labs provide this service--one in Germany, one in Greece and one in South Korea.

We Fine-Tuned Efforts

Following several years of testing, at Century Wellness we found that the Greek Test offers the most important information in terms of the number of chemotherapy agents and supplements that are tested along with the greatest accuracy.

To its credit, the Greek company, RGCC, Research Genetic Cancer Centre, tests at least 18 families of chemotherapy agents and 38 families of supplements.

Once RGCC receives the blood, the testing process takes from 10 days to two weeks for completion of the analysis. To do this, the lab's technicians and scientists sample and harvest the cancer cells--which are then cultured en vitro for gene analysis.

These specific characteristics within the patient's genes are then compared in relationship with how--if at all--the various chemotherapy agents interact with these markers. This way lab technicians determine which of the 18 specific drugs and 38 supplements work best, if any. In "hormone-driven" cancers the test identifies the best agents.

Upon completing this thorough analysis the Greek laboratory sends results to me. Then, after carefully reviewing this vital data, I construct a protocol involving a unique effective formula that marries the two most effective conventional drugs with all the best supplements. Once a patient agrees to pursue such a strategy, I often combine natural remedies and low-dose chemo to "work smart, rather than merely working hard." Small doses of insulin (5-10 units) are used to augment the low-dose chemotherapy.

Mainstream Oncologists Destroy the Body

The vast majority of advanced Stage IV cancer patients who visit conventional clinics are merely being poisoned by chemo that fails to do anything to eliminate their cancer. High-dose chemo often causes:

Chemo-brain syndrome: Commonly called "post-chemotherapy cognitive impairment," this hampers or wrecks the patient's cognitive abilities. According to the "Journal of Clinical Oncology," from 20 percent to 30 percent of people who undergo chemotherapy experience at least some form of chemo-brain syndrome. These outcomes have been so disturbing that the Journal of the National Cancer Institute has designated the condition as a real, measurable side effect. Some cancer survivors complain of a degradation of their cognitive abilities, plus decreases in their fluency and memory.

Cardiac toxicities: Sometimes called "cardiotoxicity," this condition occurs when the heart muscle sustains damage or the organ's ejection fraction reduces. These adverse characteristics, in turn, weaken the heart--which fails to adequately pump. The blood circulates with less efficiency than the organ had previously managed to accomplish consistently prior to the chemotherapy treatments. This can be measured by testing the ejection fraction (EF), which should be above 55 percent.

Peripheral neuropathies: This dreaded condition occurs

when the body's sensory nerves become damaged or diseased. The numerous adverse symptoms that vary among patients can include the impairment of organs or glands, plus a hampered ability of movement and a decrease or loss of sensation. A vast array of additional nerve-related damage sometimes occurs, depending on which portion of the body's nerves are effected.

Bone marrow suppression: Sometimes called "myelotoxicity," this adverse medical condition generates one or all of numerous highly adverse effects. Besides the potential loss of normal blood clotting, some patients experience a severe infections that result from a decrease in the white cells responsible for providing immunity. Just as destructive, another condition called "anemia" can severely hamper the essential life-giving ability of red blood cells to carry oxygen.

Generalized rashes: Often lasting from five to 20 days, or perhaps much longer, this condition can generate bothersome itchiness, bumps, cracked or blistered skin, debilitating pain, and a variety of other adverse conditions such as secondary infections due to cracks or blisters.

Death: Conventional oncologists typically prefer to avoid discussing this topic at length with patients, but there is no escaping the fact that the needless or reckless over-use of chemotherapy often results in unnecessary death. Quite predictably many patients suffer from some or even all of the previously mentioned symptoms triggered by chemo, before dying from severe levels of these adverse side effects. Most allopathic cancer doctors refrain from admitting this disturbing fact--many of their patients are killed by the highly toxic and poisonous chemo, rather than succumbing to the cancer itself.

Better Choices Available

As a licensed oncologist I'm required by law and by industry protocol to give each Stage IV cancer patient the option of having conventional high-dose chemo "treatments"--instances where such a strategy would be required of standard oncologists.

The vast majority of people with advanced-stage cancer who visit my clinic freely choose to avoid high doses of dangerous drugs. These patients usually follow my recommendation of a low-dose insulin potentiated chemo regimen, coupled with effective natural remedies--as determined by genetic testing.

For these individuals, my clinic administers low-dose fractionated insulin-potentiated regimens often referred to as "IPT." This technique "tricks the cancers" into opening up certain biological receptors. This happens due to a cancer's enhanced supply of insulin receptors. Amazingly, these are how PET scans work.

These attributes leave the cancer open to potentially effective attacks by apoptosis-producing natural Poly-MVA administered by my clinic's medical personnel. This tactic often works because cancers can only thrive on simple sugars.

As a result, the cancers often die or go into remission, robbing the disease of its ultimate goal of killing the patient.

Important Book Emerged

One of my many patients became so impressed with this process that she wrote a compelling book about her positive experience being treated at Century Wellness Clinic.

Las Vegas-based businesswoman Diana Warren chronicled her story in "Say No to Radiation and Conventional Chemo--Winning My Battle Against Stage II Breast Cancer."

Prior to visiting my office Warren had gone to numerous mainstream oncologists. All of those medical professionals had insisted that she endure high-dose chemo treatments and radiation therapy.

Brave, intelligent and charismatic, Warren refused to cave in to their dangerous medical procedures. Instead, she let common sense serve as her guide, while ignoring the reckless protocol of mainstream physicians.

Warren undertook an in-depth research regimen, eventually deciding to visit my Reno-based clinic 450 miles from Las Vegas.

Then, at my urging, Warren decided to take the "Greek Test," the chemosensitivity analysis.

The test results arrived within several weeks. Right away I worked with Warren in developing her personalized treatment regimen. We used a combination of the medications and supplements that the analysis had identified as the most effective for her body and particular type of cancer.

Warren's unique and specialized low-dose chemo treatment regimen began within several weeks at Century Wellness Clinic. Her cancer went into remission soon afterward, and at the time of this book's publication she had remained in remission for more than four and a half years before sustaining a reversible relapse.

Numerous Positive Outcomes

Although I would never refer to myself in such glowing terms, numerous doctors and industry observers refer to me as a "virtual rock star within the medical industry."

Rooms filled with Homeopaths and their assistants often erupt into applause or give standing ovations as soon as I enter some medical industry conferences.

Always in high demand to attend such functions, I usually visit from six to 10 medical industry seminars yearly throughout the United States. You see, I continually learn more about fighting cancer while always developing effective, natural ways to fight the disease.

The positive focus on me and my clinic's techniques intensified when an intelligent and highly respected celebrity, Suzanne Somers, mentioned these critical details in worldwide media forums. Somers became so impressed that she described my clinic's cancer treatment procedures in her runaway 2010 bestseller, "Knockout: Interviews With Doctors Who are Curing Cancer--And How to Prevent Getting It in the First Place."

Huge percentages of my patients learn of Century Wellness Clinic via positive word-of-mouth from other people previously treated at my clinic. Streams of my patients first learn about me in Somers' book, or from the many books that I have written, or co-authored, or from publications where other writers praise my medical procedures.

Groundbreaking Doctor Pushes the Proverbial Envelope

An internationally acclaimed Los Angeles physician and surgeon, Doctor Patrick Soon-Shiong, has generally been using the same overall type of genomic-related testing and cancer treatment that my Century Wellness Clinic has been using with much success.

With an estimated personal worth of $11 billion, Soon-Shiong has been called "a genius, a showman, an innovator and a hypster," CBS News correspondent Doctor Sanjay Gupta, said in a "60 Minutes" program segment first aired on Dec. 7, 2014.

Like me, Soon-Shiong has had his advance-stage cancer treatment methodology come into question from some mainstream doctors. Those physicians insist that more time is needed to determine if such genomic testing and low-dose treatments are effective and worthy of being recommended.

Yet as if echoing statements that I have made for several years, Soon-Shiong told Gupta that patients suffering from advance-stage cancer lack the luxury of time needed to wait for extensive testing and federal approval of new treatments.

"I'm incredibly encouraged to say that we are on the path," Soon-Shiong told "60 Minutes." "And the technology to do these things is not just hypothetical."

Soon-Shiong insists that scientists are learning to unmask cancer's molecular secrets, thanks largely to advances in DNA technology, coupled with a high-speed genome sequencing machine that he developed.

Similar to a process that I implemented at my clinic, the billionaire doctor prefers to have his advance-stage cancer patients undergo genomic testing. Like me, he strives to determine which specific drugs have the greatest probability of effectively killing the cancer of each patient.

Another similarity to my clinic's general protocol emerges

from the fact that Soon-Shiong prefers administering low-dose chemo treatments.

Similar Overall Techniques Lead to Success

In yet another significant similarity, Soon-Shiong insists that many people have a mistaken belief that cancer cells merely "grow." Instead, because of a mysterious and still-misunderstood genetic mutation, the worst cancers essentially have *the inability to die*.

In our separate, unaffiliated medical practices while still employing similar overall strategies, Soon-Shiong's clinic and mine share a mutual professional and highly focused obsession with using genomic technology to determine the characteristics of cancer's strange mutation.

Ultimately, this often results in an improved long-term survival rate, always starting with a thorough analysis of each individual patient's genomic structure and specific type of cancer.

In best-case scenarios, these advances in cancer diagnosis and treatment ultimately lead to instances where the disease becomes categorized as completely gone or when cancer evolves into a "chronic health conditions" rather than fatal.

"Overall, these advancements are clicking into gear at a far greater pace than many people realize," I sometimes tell patients. "The old way of treating cancer patients with high-dose chemo should quickly emerge as 'a thing of the past,' replaced by a much more effective era."

Century Wellness Clinic Leads the Way

Almost every day the whole world seems to be banging on my clinic's door, eager and desperate to benefit from substantial advances in genomic technology.

Yet amazingly only an infinitesimal fraction of the 7 billion living people worldwide knows that my clinic uses these amazing anti-cancer techniques.

My office doors are always open weekdays, except on a handful of U.S. holidays and during the brief span from Christmas through New Year's Day.

As you might very well imagine, my office phones are continually "ringing off the hook" while people ask for appointments.

Many patients tell me that they're pleased and delighted upon discovering that my staff is eager to answer any questions that they might have.

Demand Continues to Intensify

The patient load at Century Wellness Clinic continues on a steady increase. Every step of the way we strive to make the process as stress-free and easy as possible for each person eager for an examination and treatment.

I have already stated the following in the first chapter, but I need to re-emphasize the details here because the important facts are essential to all my patients:

Many people vising for the first time admit they're impressed by the fact that nearly two-thirds of my Stage IV cancer patients remain alive and in remission from the disease--6 years after their initial treatments at Century Wellness Clinic.

Remember, this means that six out of every 10 worst-stage cancer patients that I treat remain alive, most relatively healthy and capable of enjoying life to the fullest.

By contrast, according to numerous nationwide medical reports, only two out of every 100 Stage IV cancer patients survive when treated by mainstream oncologists.

So, knowing these details, who would you choose--the doctors required to administer high-dose poison in all such cases, or me, an expert at administering an effective combination of low-dose chemo, natural remedies and healthy supplements?

Take These Important Steps

To help optimize results and make their excursions as stress-free as possible, all first-time patients visiting Century Wellness Clinic can:

Call: 775-827-0707, or toll free 877-789-0707; tell the receptionist your health situation, so that we can start the process of potentially making a reservation.

Records: Upon making a reservation, you must bring copies of your records from your current doctor, or send us that information before arriving. This information should include any and all available reports regarding oncology, pathology, surgery, chemotherapy, X-rays, scans, laboratory tests, narrative summaries, and a list of all medications and supplements.

Frailty: Like all doctors, we generally are unable to treat patients who have become "extremely frail;" under this condition the person's body mass and weight have dropped to precipitously low levels--while muscles have nearly disappeared.

Prior Treatments: Preferably before their first visit to Century Wellness, patients should avoid being treated elsewhere by mainstream oncologists. The high-dose chemo and radiation administered by those doctors seriously weakens and damages the body--thereby decreasing the potential effectiveness of subsequent treatments. Homeopaths refer to people with cancer who refrain from chemo and radiation prior to visiting doctors of natural medicine as "virginal treatment patients." Although we prefer treating "virginal patients," in many instances my clinic accepts people with cancer who already have been treated by conventional oncologists. In order to be accepted, such candidates must communicate with a member of my staff before a decision is made.

Travel & Accommodations: New and returning patients make their own arrangements for travel and lodging. The Reno area has numerous high-quality hotels and restaurants at mid-range and high-end prices. Car rentals via Reno-Tahoe International Airport are available for those who travel by air, and shuttle services are provided by most major hotel-casinos in the region.

Location: Century Wellness Clinic is at 521 Hammill Lane in South Reno, an ideal site just one block from on-ramps and off-ramps to U.S. Interstate 580--one of the region's two primary highways. A north-south arterial, I-580 provides easy access to the airport, all of the region's primary hotels, and the region's primary east-west highway, U.S. Interstate 80. Travel time to or from the airport and the clinic is about 10 minutes.

Activities: During "free" time when not undergoing medical examinations or treatments, patients, their relatives or friends have a vast array of options for fun, relaxing, energizing or restful activities. The high-desert region surrounding Reno, which is at 4,500 feet above sea level, has hundreds of miles of hiking trails providing panoramic views. The city is just a one-hour drive from Lake Tahoe, an ideal summer playground. Nestled in the Sierra at 6,200 feet above sea level, as North America's largest alpine lake, Tahoe has easy access to dozens of ski resorts popular during winter. Just as enticing, the historic Comstock Lode mining town of Virginia City, where the legendary writer Mark Twain began his journalism career for the "Territorial Enterprise" in the 1860s, is just a 30-minute drive southeast of Reno. Virginia City has numerous popular attractions including museums, and historic saloons such as the the world famous Bucket of Blood saloon.

Expected stays: Patients visiting for initial examinations and chemosensitivity testing usually stay from several days to one week. Those undergoing treatment regimens of low-dose chemo, effective natural remedies and supplements usually stay from two to three weeks. Subsequent visits for standard examinations are usually recommended for patients who have undergone treatments, so that I can monitor each person's progress in beating cancer. Follow-up visits for examinations usually are arranged in three- or six-month, or one-year intervals; these spans hinge on the type of cancer a patient had, the current suspected severity of the disease; and whether the cancer has gone into--or seems to progressing into--remission.

Additional treatment: Some patients occasionally require or request follow-up treatment regimens if their cancer remains active following the initial round.

Various ailments: Century Wellness Clinic treats patients suffering from many types of ailments, particularly cancer. We treat all types of the disease in any bodily area and at every level of severity; besides advanced Stage IV cancer, the clinic treats patients suffering from less severe levels including Stage II and Stage III. Patients need to know that unless effectively treated all types of cancer can worsen to the dreaded Stage IV; the worst-stage cancers invariably lead to death unless successfully treated. In addition, many patients learn prior to their initial visits to Century Wellness that mainstream oncologists strive to administer poisonous and deadly high-dose chemo to patients suffering from the less severe Stage II or Stage III levels of the disease--not just Stage IV.

Critical Patient Choices

Keep in mind that as previously stated, throughout every phase of each patient's examinations and treatment I give the patient the option of making critical choices.

This marks a sharp contrast from the style of mainstream oncologists, who essentially say without using such specific words: "It's my way, or the highway."

I give each patient the option of receiving natural remedies that are proven highly effective, always with the patient's physical and mental well-being in mind.

In doing so, I'm essentially following the philosophy of Doctor Benjamin Rush, a signer of the Declaration of Independence and the personal physician of U.S. President George Washington.

"Unless we put medical freedom into the Constitution, the time will come when medicine will organize into an undercover dictatorship," said Rush, a founding father of the United States who died in 1813 at age 67. "To restrict the art of healing to one class of men and deny equal privileges to others will cause a Bastille of medical science.

"All such laws are un-American and despotic, and have no place in a republic. The Constitution of this republic should make a special privilege for medical freedom."

To the detriment of all types of patients, no such provisions were included in the USA's founding documents. Since then mainstream doctors have run roughshod over patients' rights; these physicians have used their political allies to implement and control federal agencies that require or sanction the use of ineffective, costly, and poisonous deadly drugs.

Whole Body and Soul

Effectively treating patients can only happen when addressing the whole body, the mind and what I sometimes call the person's "positive spirit or soul."

Unlike mainstream oncologists who poison the entire body in an effort "to fix an isolated cancer," I incorporate a whole-body strategy using mostly natural remedies.

Besides administering low-dose chemo with natural remedies, personnel at my clinic also help address numerous issues in order to improve each patient's overall health. Among these critical health-enhancing tactics that mainstream oncologists ignore are:

Balance: We show each patient how to achieve a balanced lifestyle using an ideal combination of rest, exercise, sleep, nutrition and activities suited for emotional harmony.

Detoxify: Clean the body of foreign or unnatural substances that are likely to damage overall health, while sometimes also sometimes triggering cancer.

Diet: The common saying that "you are what you eat" remains true, sometimes leading to cancer due to unhealthy diets. So, we teach patients about good nutrition.

Empower: As previously stated, we give each patient choices about treatment, recovery and strategies to achieve or to maintain optimal health.

Information: We teach patients the critical details that they must know to detect, prevent and control cancer.

Sugar: We teach each patient that common sugars, particular when ingested in high amounts, are a leading cause of cancer--which "love and thrives" on this substance.

Supplements: Use the supplements identified by

chemosensitivity testing as the most helpful for a specific cancer patient; these products contain vitamins, minerals and various herbs. They serve as the backbone for good overall physical, mental and spiritual health.

Target Specific Cancers

I have developed unique, individualized strategies to effectively battle each form of cancer.

This is unlike mainstream oncologists who--as previously stated--use an ill-advised and ineffective "one-size-fits-all" approach to almost every form of the disease.

By analyzing an individual's chemosensitivity test, physical examination and medical records, I'm able to marry the best natural remedies in combination with low-dose chemo, along with supplements identified as the most effective for the person.

Doctors classify each form of cancer based on the bodily area where the disease started. Compounding the challenge, each type of cancer has a unique growth rate, pattern of spreading and response to specific treatments.

Many physicians and particularly Homeopaths have deemed me as perhaps the world's premiere expert at developing and matching the ideal and most effective treatment for each type of cancer.

Chemosensitivity tests are particularly helpful because each person has a unique, one-of-a-kind genomic structure unlike any other person.

Risk Factors Play a Role

Intense and continuous worldwide genomic research has been identifying and confirming what many physicians have suspected for a long time.

Genomic research has confirmed that some individuals have a greater likelihood than the general population of developing specific types of cancer.

For instance, women from some families have a far greater

chance of developing breast cancer than most females throughout the general population.

At least some good news has emerged. Scientists have confirmed that the inherited probability of cancer is less prevalent than previously thought.

As a result, some researchers and medical facilities have informally categorized most cancer causes as instances where the individual is a victim of "bad luck."

Many severe risk factors sharply increase the probability of getting cancer. Besides smoking or chewing tobacco, these include exposure to chemicals, ultraviolet light, free radicals in foods, red or processed meats, sugar, air pollution and many more.

In addition, each specific risk factor increases a person's chances of getting certain cancers. For instance, smoking or chewing tobacco sharply increases a person's risk of developing cancers of the lung, tongue, mouth, larynx, and other organs. Scientists blame most skin cancers on excessive exposure to the sun or suntanning machines.

Most tumors are benign or lacking cancer; such tumors are usually non-threatening, except in rare exceptions.

In all instances of cancer, a person's chances of "being cured" increase drastically the sooner the disease is discovered and treated; cancers that are allowed to grow and spread over extended periods without being treated sharply increase the chances of developing into deadly advanced Stage IV levels of the disease.

My War in Fighting Cancer

In the fight against cancer, patients at Century Wellness Clinic might think of me as a proverbial five-star general or a commander-in-chief.

Under my continual command the clinic's staff administers at least 17 strategies, many that I have personally designed to destroy cancer. With added importance, some of these strategies strive to put each patient on a pathway toward optimal overall health.

Besides the unique chemosensitivity testing of whole blood, one of these key techniques briefly mentioned earlier involves the low-dose fractionated regimens sometimes called "IPT."

As previously stated, when using a unique system that I personally developed, the process strives to "trick" or "fool" the disease into opening certain receptors within the cancer's cells. This happens in part because cancers desperately crave energy-producing sugar and thrive in low-dose and acidic tissues.

I work to ensure that this natural process opens biological receptors. When this happens the cancer is left wide-open to horrific attacks, while the rest of the body remains unharmed and safe.

The typical weaponry that I employ here involves a natural substance, the harmless and effective Poly-MVA expertly administered by my staff. This is usually done on alternate days with low-dose fractionated chemotherapy, levels much smaller and far less harmful to the body than chemo typically administered by mainstream oncologists.

Napoleonic Battles Against Cancer

Although despotic, often cruel and heartless, the famed French Emperor and my clinic treats people with other health issues that compromise or weaken immunity.

Biological Response Modifiers: Besides the immune enhancement technique listed immediately above, we also employ "biological response modifiers" that are sometimes called "BRMs." Remember that as mentioned earlier, the effective strategies that I employ typically strive to kill at least 90 percent of a patient's cancer, and from that point the person's immune system plays a critical role in fighting and successfully killing the remainder of the disease. Similar to substances naturally produced by the body and often created by scientists in laboratories, BRMs super-charge the body's natural response to infection and to cancer. This "immunotherapy" treatment process enhances the body's immune systems, particularly natural defenses against cancer. Also, because my clinic serves patients with ailments other than cancer, we sometimes use BRMs to affectively address such adverse conditions as rheumatoid arthritis. Although comprised of natural substances, the administering of BRMs on extremely rare occasion generates adverse symptoms such as diarrhea, nausea, vomiting and loss of appetite. Thus, BRMs should only be taken in a professional medical environment that monitors patients.

Bio-Oxidative Therapy: A super-powerful tool among natural healing methods, the natural process called "bio-oxidative therapy" serves as a stong anti-oxidant and cancer killer. Unlike humans and all mammals, cancer gets its oxygen from the fermentation process, rather than breathing from the environment. At my recommendation and upon patient approval, I use bio-oxidative therapy to surround cancer cells with oxygen. This high-oxygen environment can significantly decrease the disease's ability to grow and to divide. Meantime, this therapy typically stimulates receptors in white blood cells, thus boosting the immune system and fortifying the body's natural strength and effectiveness in attacking cancer. Perhaps just as impressive, this therapy increases the body's natural production of interferon, interleukin-2 and tumor necrosis factor--all factors that sharply boost the body's natural cancer fighting processes. Meantime, bio-oxidative therapy also often improves the health of patients who have been ill, thanks to the ability of this process to increase oxygen tension in bodily tissues.

Lifestyle guidance: Clinic staff members often teach or suggest ways for an individual patient to enjoy life to the fullest extent possible. Such positive behavioral changes often make the person feel better both physically and emotionally, thereby decreasing the likelihood that a cancer will worsen or return. When giving this advice, my personnel consider numerous simultaneous factors including the person's type and severity of cancer, level of remission, overall health, and all other ailments currently experienced by the individual.

Professional referrals: As a highly experienced doctor with extensive medical industry contacts throughout Northern Nevada and worldwide, I sometimes refer patients who need additional services to other medical professionals ranging from surgeons to radiologists.

Second opinions: After initially receiving the diagnosis of physicians elsewhere, some people visit Century Wellness Clinic to seek a "second opinion" from me and other doctors on my staff. Sometimes we reach similar conclusions, although in numerous instances either I or my personnel generate findings that differ from what the patient had been told elsewhere.

Coping skills: Century Wellness Clinic offers individual and group counseling, unlike the vast majority of mainstream oncologists and cancer treatment facilities nationwide. At my clinic, skilled advisers highly knowledgeable in medicine and optimal lifestyles teach patients or their families how to cope and excel in key issues. Patients and their families learn optimal ways to administer effective healthcare, plus suggested methods on handling daily lifestyle tasks or personal responsibilities.

l Napoléon Bonaparte of the early 19th Century remains world-famous for his dastardly war tactics of suddenly attacking enemies using extreme unconventional tactics.

At least within the realm of battling cancer, many of my patients think of me as using "Napoleonic battle plans against the disease within the practices of both oncology and Homeopathy."

Highly detailed books could be separately written and published about each of my most popular and effective cancer-fighting strategies. Besides chemosensitivity tests, IPT, and low-dose fractionated chemotherapy, here is a brief summary of some of the most effective methods frequently used at Century Wellness Clinic:

Healthful water: Because healthful, pure water can boost energy while ridding the body of harmful and potentially cancerous impurities, we provide patients with access to "alkaline H2O pH therapy." The water is at an optimal alkaline level, the opposite from the harmful acidic range. This strategy serves an important role because cancer thrives within an acidic environment; the pH levels of cancer patients are typically far more acidic than alkaline.

Nutritional guidance: What a person chooses to eat plays a critical role in either generating or preventing cancer. Many of these "poor" and "good" choices hinge on whether a particular food is within the healthful alkaline or unhealthy acidic ranges. We show patients meal plans developed for their unique personal situations. These details can be found in my book, the "Forsythe Anti-Cancer Diet;" it's available in paper or e-reader form via all major bookstores and online eBook venues.

Individualized nutrition: Besides the advice on diet briefly mentioned above, we develop cancer-fighting and cancer-preventing regimens that include specific foods, vitamins, and herbs. As I often tell patients, natural substances such as these generally are far more preferable than unnatural or synthetic drugs typically administered by mainstream oncologists. Besides helping to boost overall health, such products serve as just one of the many ways that we help give the body a fighting, natural chance against cancer.

Immune Enhancement: Cancer typically compromises or wrecks the body's immune system, often robbing the person of energy and the ability to fight the disease. To counteract this detrimental condition, we administer a high-dose Vitamin-C immune booster that patients receive intravenously as a standard procedure. Often loaded with vital additional vitamins and supplements, these immune-enhancing sessions often sharply increase the body's natural ability to battle certain ailments-- particularly cancer.

Patients Deserve Priority Status

At Century Wellness Clinic, every patient gets "priority status;" they all deserve and receive respect without being ignored or told, "Do this and do that. Take this poison, because you have no other choice."

The doctors and personnel at my facility strongly embrace this highly coveted mission statement. We strive to show each patient that the clinic truly cares, while effectively working in an effort to achieve the best possible results.

Blessed with a keen knowledge of the art and science of medicine, I continually draw upon all treatment modalities ranging from the most advanced conventional therapies to mainstream medicine. All along, I also incorporate the most effective remedies of Homeopathic medicine, primarily natural therapies ignored by mainstream oncologists.

Using these medical systems as a solid foundation for giving all patients the best possible care, I have developed four options uniquely designed to fulfill their desires:

One: Fractionated conventional chemotherapy alone

Two: Fractional low-dose chemotherapy, plus Homeopathic treatments including Insulin Potentiated Therapy (IPT)

Three: Complimentary Homeopathic and/or naturopathic modalities alone

Four: Best supportive therapy

Based on my intensive studies, I have discovered that superior results occur when using combination treatments of: fractionated (low-dose) chemotherapy; Homeopathic intravenous remedies; and immune-stimulating supplements including organic herbs.

Along with my staff throughout the course of treating thousands of patients, I have developed intense studies on: Paw-Paw, a naturally grown substance deemed highly effective in cancer treatment; Poly-MVA, a uniquely formulated combination of minerals and amino acids designed to support cellular energy and promote overall good health, while also highly effective for treating cancer; the Forsythe Immune Protocol, a highly effective immune-enhancing process that I personally developed to significantly boost positive results in the treatment of my cancer patients; and a combination of the Forsythe Immune Protocol, CST and IPT.

A "Bill of Rights" for Patients

Determined to counteract the "dogmatic rules" imposed by mainstream oncologists who refuse to allow patients to make vital choices regarding their own health, I have developed an essential "Bill of Rights" that all people with cancer can embrace. Among some of the most important proclamations:

Positive attitude: Each patient has a right to refrain from becoming afraid or discouraged, always cognizant that at various times in recent years medical literature has chronicled cures for all types of cancer.

Alternative path: Patients have a right to chose a unique, extremely rare integrative medical oncologist such as me because I'm highly skilled at treating their entire bodies with harmless and effective natural remedies--plus drugs when necessary.

High-dose chemo: Patients have a right to refuse extensive high-dose chemo regimens that mainstream oncologists insist on administering. When and if such a refusal is made, the patient should have a right to seek out the services of an extremely rare integrative medical oncologist such as me--capable of administering effective natural remedies.

Remain skeptical: Patients have a right to "keep an open mind about issues," while also remaining skeptical when reading or hearing about the supposed results of various clinical studies--particularly instances where two or more drugs are used.

Show spunk: Each patient has a right to peacefully "stand his or her own ground" as a self-preservation measure. Such instances might involve politely leaving an oncologist's office when the doctor mentions "hospice care" or "getting your affairs in order." Such statements indicate that the physician has given up on you; all patients have a right to embrace an attitude that: "I will never give up on myself."

Food choices: Patients have a right and a responsibility to themselves to adopt good eating habits, following the advice of their Homeopaths, physicians and dietitians.

Avoid unnecessary tests: Patients have a right to refuse over-testing, particularly procedures that involve radiation; radiological scans that target various areas of the body's overall immune system are particularly dangerous. Such procedures endanger overall health, increasing the likelihood that immune defenses will fail to work at optimal levels.

Alternative medicines: Patients have a right to know about, to use and to benefit from effective natural remedies that mainstream oncologists refuse to mention or to use. Of particular importances are beneficial supplements that often emerge as extremely helpful and essential in fighting cancer; supplements also eliminate carcinogens and toxins from the body.

Beware of media: Patients have a right and a responsibility to themselves to remain wary of advertisements or promotions that strive to fool them. For instance, some cancer centers claim to have the latest "pinpointed radiology procedures."

Refuse certain surgeries: Particularly among those with advanced Stage IV cancer, patients have a right to avoid a doctor's insistence that they undergo aggressive surgical procedures. These include second-look operations and devastating head-and-neck surgeries requiring tracheotomy and/or gastric feeding tubes.

Limit drugs: Patients have a right to limit the amount of drugs that they take. Whenever possible a patient should be able to take the smallest number of drugs, administered at the lowest-possible doses needed to fight their cancer. This strategy can minimize or prevent the destruction of the person's vital immune system.

Patients Praise Me

I receive heart-felt, compelling and emotional letters or emails each week from all over the world, sent by patients extremely grateful for their improved health.

"I'm so grateful to remain alive," is a phrase signifying a common theme. "I'm eternally grateful for the new lease on life that you have given me."

Some of my now-healthy former patients retell their stories, recounting the fact that they had previously been told elsewhere that: "You are going to die."

Imagine being informed that you are definitely going to be killed within a certain limited number of weeks or months, only to subsequently learn after finally being treated by me that you are going to live.

While glad to receive these messages, I refrain from dwelling on them--partly due to the need to continually concentrate on my job of "saving" as many people as possible.

Of course, not all of my patients survive. Yet as previously stated, the five-year survival rate of my advanced Stage IV cancer patients is far greater than the national average. Remember, according to my clinic's current study involving 1,000 patients, only two out of every 100 Stage IV cancer patients treated by mainstream oncologists survive, while at least 71 of such people that I treat remain alive at six years.

Essential Details

As previously mentioned, even following my success in treating cancer patients, I never can, have or will issue any guarantee that any patient will be cured or experience a significant improvement in his or her overall medical condition.

With this clearly understood, readers should remain fully cognizant of the fact that the details that I have provided in this book are strictly for educational and informational purposes only.

In addition, you should refrain from considering any or all statements that I have made here as medical advice--specifically because at this point we can assume that you are not yet a patient of mine.

I only make specific diagnosis and issue recommendations individually to each of my patients after conducting a thorough physical examination and reviewing medical records.

With these "disclaimer" factors clearly understood,

my clinic welcomes inquiries from potential patients. Also, prospective patients should know that Century Wellness Clinic, also known as the Forsythe Cancer Care Center, is an out-patient facility without overnight accommodations.

Bibliography
Nanorobots Use Bee Venom to Battle Cancer
http://tinyurl.com/BeeVenomTargetsCancer
Nanobees Might Become Popular Worldwide
http://tinyurl.com/NanobeeBenefits
Hospitals consider robots
http://tinyurl.com/HospitalsConsiderRobots
Nurses and Robotics
http://preview.tinyurl.com/NursesAndRobotics
Physicians Say Robots Will Help
http://tinyurl.com/RoboDocIssue
Robots Enter Hospitals
http://tinyurl.com/RobotsEnterHospitals
Imaging Technology News on why robots can replace doctors
http://tinyurl.com/RoboticImaging
Medical Robot Critics Express Concerns
http://tinyurl.com/MedicalRobotCritics
Association of American Medical Colleges Issues Warning
http://tinyurl.com/HumanDoctorsFaceChallenges
Obamacare Threatens Doctors
http://tinyurl.com/ObamacareThreatensDoctors
General public envisions profound technological change
http://tinyurl.com/PublicOpinionTechnology
Experts predict 30 percent of jobs will be automated by 2025
http://tinyurl.com/2025JobLosses
Oxford University predicts 47 percent of jobs lost to robots by 2035
http://tinyurl.com/2035JobLosses
Finding jobs in China becomes major issue due to robots
http://tinyurl.com/ChinaJobHuntIssue
Musk, Gates, Wozniak, and Hawking issue warning
http://tinyurl.com/MuskGatesHawkingWozniak
Robots Endanger More Jobs
http://tinyurl.com/RobotsEndangerMoreJobs
Forbes article stresses little impact from robots
http://tinyurl.com/OpinionOnJobLosses

Forecast: University and College Foreclosures Will Triple
http://tinyurl.com/UniversityCollegeClosuresTripl
University of Phoenix closes more than 100 campuses
http://tinyurl.com/PhoenixUniversityClosures
Federal Agency, Darpa, planting microchips in human brains
http://tinyurl.com/DarpaImplantingChips
Scientists Use Microchips to Boost Monkey Intelligence
http://tinyurl.com/MonkeyIntelligenceBoosted
Robotic Brain Discoveries Accelerate
http://tinyurl.com/RoboticBrainDiscoveries
Advancements Undermine Human Experience
http://tinyurl.com/UndermineHumanExperience
History's First Official Robot Marriage
http://tinyurl.com/RobotMarriesPerson
Scholarly Article on Robotic Relationships
http://tinyurl.com/ScholarlyRoboticRelationships
Human-Robot Relationship Ethics
http://tinyurl.com/HumanRobotEthics
Humans Place Too Much Trust in Robots
http://tinyurl.com/HumansTrustRobotsTooMuch
Charles Schwab Launches Schwab Intelligent Portfolios
https://intelligent.schwab.com/
"Wired" magzine reports advances in medical robotics
programming
http://tinyurl.com/MedicalProgrammingAdvances
"Fusion" magazine reports advancements in speed-writing
http://tinyurl.com/RoboJournalism
"PC Magazine:" Dell has developed computer-based cognitive
intelligence
http://tinyurl.com/ComputerBasedRobotics
Scientists develop robotic brain cells
http://tinyurl.com/RobotBrainCells
"Tech Republic" analysis of Google robotics shopping spree
http://tinyurl.com/GoogleBuyingRobots
"The Verge" reports that Boston Dynmics robots have mind-

blowing capabilities
http://tinyurl.com/BostonDynamicsRobots
"Popular Science" analyzes Google's move into robotics
http://tinyurl.com/PopularScienceAnalyzeGoogle
Inverse Magazine describes "Franksetin Complex," Extreme Fear of Robots
http://tinyurl.com/RoboticFears
"The Naked Ape" book by Desmond Morris
http://tinyurl.com/TheNakedApeBook
"Irish Examiner" article discussed the hacking of robots
http://tinyurl.com/RobotHackingDiscussed
"Western Journalism" publication reveals Obamacare database flaws
http://tinyurl.com/ObamacareDatabaseFlaws
"Forbes Magazine" chronicles the hacker culture
http://tinyurl.com/ForbesDiscussesHackers
"Huffington Post" reports that AI will generate income inequaltiy
http://tinyurl.com/HuffingtonAI
"International Business Times" on medical robots with AI
http://tinyurl.com/IntBizTimesAI
"The Guardian" Chronicles AI Issues
http://tinyurl.com/TheGuardianOnAI
"Inverse Magazine" commentary and article on AI
http://tinyurl.com/InverseOnAI
"Tech Times" Reports on First Fully Digital Hospital in North America
http://tinyurl.com/TechTimesDigitalHospital
"Market Watch" report on Artificial Ingelligence
http://tinyurl.com/MarketWatchAI
"Gov Insider" report on AI
http://tinyurl.com/GovInsiderPI
"PC World" report on AI app
http://tinyurl.com/PCWorldAIApp
"Fast Company" on satellites using AI to monitor poverty
http://tinyurl.com/FastCompanyAISatellites

"International Business Times:" AI used to help blind people
http://tinyurl.com/InternationalBusinessTimesAI
"Portland Press Herald" article by "Washington Post" on AI in toys
http://tinyurl.com/PortlandPressHearldAI
"MIT Technology Review" on whether medical robotics will increase patient costs
http://tinyurl.com/MITCostReview
"Lifelong Health" on the costs of medical robots
http://tinyurl.com/LifelongHealthRobots
"HFM Magazine" on medical robotics cost benefits
http://tinyurl.com/HFMagazineBenefits
American Society of Mechanical Engineers on medical robot costs
http://tinyurl.com/ASMEcostAnalysis
"Mother Nature Network" on technological dependance
http://tinyurl.com/MotherNatureNetworkTech
"Daily Mail" on Telepresence Robots in classrooms
http://tinyurl.com/DailyMailTeachingRobots
"The Street" analysis of robotics industry
http://tinyurl.com/TheStreetRobotStocks
"Investor Place" on medical robotics stocks
http://tinyurl.com/InvestorPlaceRoboticsStocks
"Medical Robotics Magazine" description
http://tinyurl.com/MedicalRoboticsMagazine
"San Diego Union Tribune" on robotics club challenges
http://tinyurl.com/SanDiegoUnionRobots
"Goshen News" on robotics in classrooms
http://tinyurl.com/GoshenNewsOnRobotics
"Dickson County News" on robots for trash disposal
http://tinyurl.com/DicksonCountyNewsTrash
"The Monitor" on After School Robotics Clubs
http://tinyurl.com/TheMonitorAfterSchoolClubs
"News Observer" on high school's new robotics club
http://tinyurl.com/NewsObserverRobotClub
NBC News on Universities helping NASA develop robots

http://tinyurl.com/NBCNewsRobotics
"Daily Courier" on Robotics Clubs in Arizona
http://tinyurl.com/DailyCourierRobots
"Weather Network" on university students monitoring NASA's
Mars Robots
http://tinyurl.com/WeatherNetworkNASArobots
"Run Direct Magazine" on military robot production rate
http://tinyurl.com/RunDirectMagazineMilitaryRobot
"WhaTech" report on the spread of military robots
http://tinyurl.com/WhaTechMilitaryRobots
"Korea Times" on robots that detect and remove mines
http://tinyurl.com/KoreaTimesMineDetection
"Tech Times" on stopping killer robots
http://tinyurl.com/TechTimesStoppingKillerRobots
"CNBC" on why people should refrain from fearing job losses
http://tinyurl.com/zrufvdv

Publications Meet Intensifying Demand

A steadily growing cadre of publications have been launched in an effort to meet demand for information from physicians and others interested in medical robotics.

Among the most widely publicized of these publications are:

"Journal of Medical Robotics Research:" A "World Scientific" report describes this publication by saying that "Medical robotics has been progressively revolutionizing treatment for at least the past two decades. The 'Journal of Medical Robotics Research' invites fundamental contributions to all areas of medical robotics including clinical evaluation studies. The journal is primarily aimed toward bringing the scientific and technological developments--as well as clinical evaluation studies--in the area of medical robotics to a wider robotics and clinical audience."

"The International Journal of Medical Robotics and Computer Assisted Surgery:" Available via all major booksellers, according to the Online Library at Wiley.com, this publication features a wide varity of in-depth articles on such technologies.

"Medical Robotics Magazine:" According to at least one blog report, this publication was founded in 2007 by John J. Otrompke. Dedicated to all aspects of the medical robotics industry, this publication features copyrighted articles on robotics surgery, and various "other topics related to robotics medicine."

"Medical Robotics:" A textbook for undergraduates in computer science and engineering, this publication Springer--released in October 2015 by Achim Schweikard and Floris Ernst--is described by the Amazon bookselling service as providing a "thorough background to the emerging field of medical robots. It covers the mathematics needed to understand the use of robotic devices in medicine, including but not limited to robot kinematics, hand-eye and robot-world calibration, reconstruction, registration, motion planning, motion prediction, motion correlation, motion replication, and Motion Learni

About the Author

James W. Forsythe, M.D., H.M.D., has long been considered one of the most respected physicians in the United States, particularly for his treatment of cancer and the legal use of human growth hormone. In the mid-1960s, Dr. Forsythe graduated with honors from University California at Berkeley and earned his Medical Degree from University of California, San Francisco, before spending two years residency in Pathology at Tripler Army Hospital, Honolulu. After a tour of duty in Vietnam, he returned to San Francisco and completed an internal medicine residency and an oncology fellowship. He is also a world-renowned speaker and author. He has co-authored, been mentioned in and/or written chapters in bestsellers. To name a few: "Stoned ~ The Truth About Medical Marijuana and Hemp Oil;" "The Human Genome Playbook for Disrupting Cancer;" "An Alternative Medicine Definitive Guide to Cancer;" "Knockout, Interviews with Doctors who are Curing Cancer" Suzanne Somers' number one bestseller; "The Ultimate Guide To Natural Health, Quick Reference A-Z Directory of Natural Remedies for Diseases and Ailments;" "Anti-Aging Cures;" "The Healing Power of Sleep;" and "Compassionate Oncology ~ What Conventional Cancer Specialists Don't Want You To Know;" and "Obaminable Care," "Complete Pain," "Natural Pain Killers," and "Your Secret to the Fountain of Youth ~ What They Don't Want You to Know About HGH Human Growth Hormone," "Take Control of Your Cancer," "Understanding and Surviving Obamacare," "About Death from a Cancer Doctor's Perspective," "Dr. Forsythe's Whey Protein Anti-Aging Formula," and the "Emergency Radiation Medical Handbook."

Contact Information

Dr. James W. Forsythe, M.D., H.M.D.
Century Wellness Clinic
521 Hammill Lane, Reno, NV 89511-1004
775-827-0707
Website: DrForsythe.com
Email: RenoWellnessDr @ yahoo.com

www.ingramcontent.com/pod-product-compliance
Lightning Source LLC
Chambersburg PA
CBHW060319200326
41519CB00011BA/1779